THE KETO GUIDO COOKBOOK

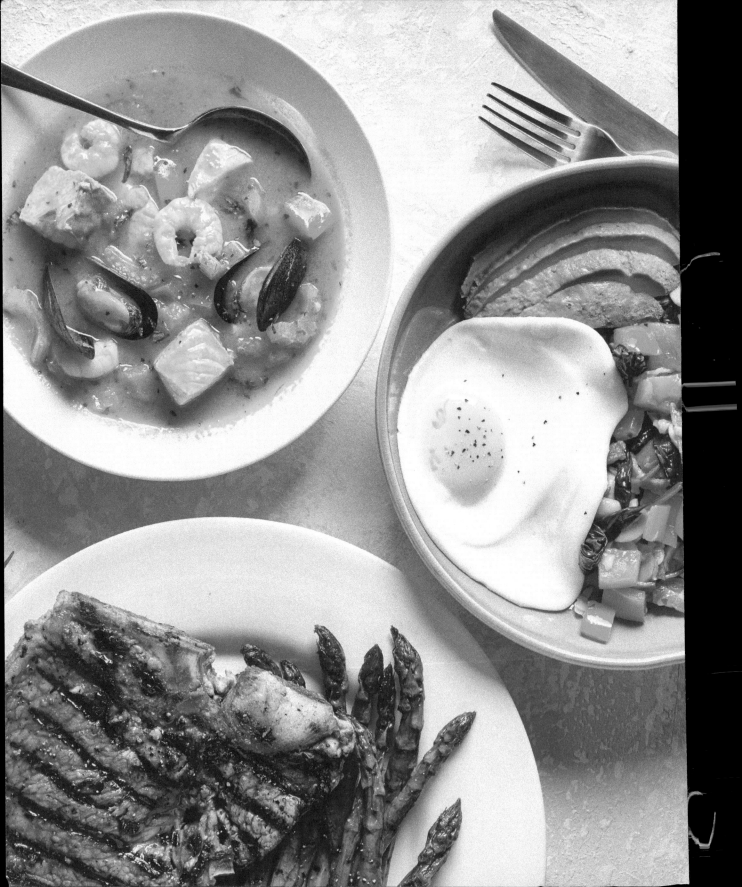

THE KETO GUIDO
COOKBOOK

DELICIOUS RECIPES TO GET HEALTHY AND LOOK GREAT

Vinny Guadagnino

ROCKRIDGE
PRESS

For general information on our other products and services or to obtain technical support, please contact our Customer Care Department within the United States at (866) 744-2665, or outside the United States at (510) 253-0500.

Rockridge Press publishes its books in a variety of electronic and print formats. Some content that appears in print may not be available in electronic books, and vice versa.

Cover Designer: Kristine Brogno
Interior Designer: Jami Spittler
Photo Art Director / Art Manager: Amy Burditt
Editor: Pippa White
Production Editor: Ashley Polikoff

Cover Photography and pp. viii -1, 6, 17 & 24 © 2019 Christoper Kern. All other interior photography © 2019 Darren Muir, except pg. 102 © Shutterstock / thefoodphotographer & pg. 173 © Nadine Greeff.

ISBN: Print 978-1-64152-482-7
eBook 978-1-64152-483-4

R1

CONTENTS

INTRODUCTION

By Paola Guadagnino

My son Vinny has been exceeding his mother's expectations ever since his earliest years. He did well in school and had plans to become a lawyer. He even studied for the LSAT exam just before landing a role on *Jersey Shore*. He had to make a choice then about the path he was going to take, and while some people might assume he took the easier path, I can tell you that being a TV personality isn't as easy as it looks. During the filming of *Jersey Shore*, Vinny experienced some anxiety. He was only 21 when they started, and he was not used to being in the spotlight and having his every move analyzed and judged. Yet he used this obstacle to propel himself forward. He spent time working on managing his anxiety, and even wrote a book about his personal experience to give his fans some of the self-help tools that he had learned.

Additionally, through Vinny's personal evolution and his effort to moderate the lifestyle that came along with being a *Jersey Shore* cast member, he became more conscious of his diet and of how he was treating his body. This led him to try the keto lifestyle, and he's never looked back. Through focus and diligence, he committed to a healthy way of eating, and made me proud once again.

You might not know it, but Vinny is a very determined and positive person. When he made the change in his diet, he did it with a lot of thought. He said to me, "In order to have a healthy mind, you need a healthy and clean body." I am proud of my son for always striving to overcome obstacles and be the best version of himself.

Even though I taught Vinny to cook, I admit that through his keto journey, he's been the one to teach me some tips along the way. I still love to cook for Vinny, so he's broadened my repertoire of ingredients. For example, I now use almond flour to make Vinny's pizza, and I've learned how to reduce my sugar intake. And all of the food we make together tastes great! As an Italian mama, I have been surprised by how much I love the low-carb meals we make. All of this comes from Vinny's hard work and research about the keto diet.

On a more personal note, I have had to accept that my Sunday pasta dinners and some other recipes had to change (well, I still get to feed him my chicken cutlets and pasta when he cheats once in a while!). Overall though, I believe that these changes have been for the best. Learning a new approach to cooking and

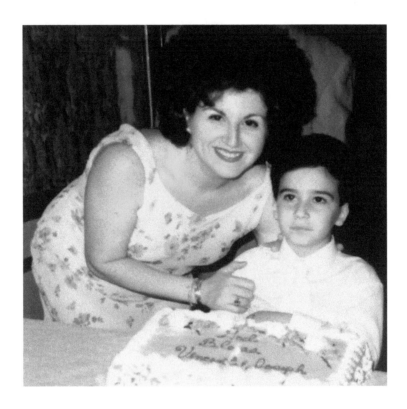

meal prepping is not only useful in the kitchen, but it's also a fun and instructive way to bond with others over food. And there's nothing more Italian than that!

Just in the way he shared his journey into keto with me, my son is now sharing the keto lifestyle with you—in this book. From a mother's point of view, it's really satisfying to see that when my son discovers something he takes a strong interest in, he wants to share it with the world. This speaks volumes about Vinny's character. His generosity truly inspires me.

I am so proud of my beautiful boy and his success in achieving his goals, but I am most proud of his desire to help others.

I hope you enjoy Vinny's meals as much as I do and get a lot out of this book!

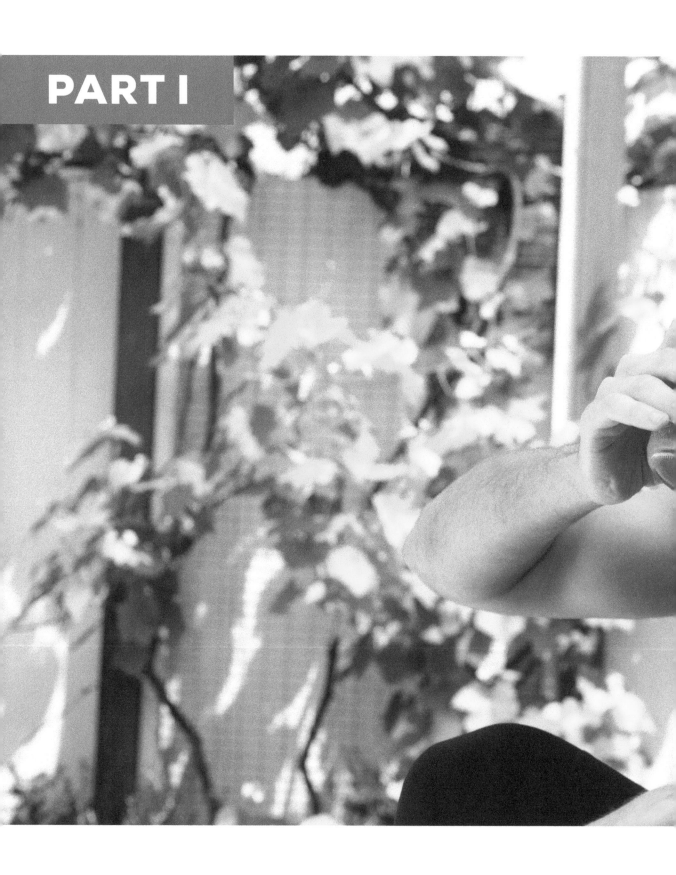

PART I

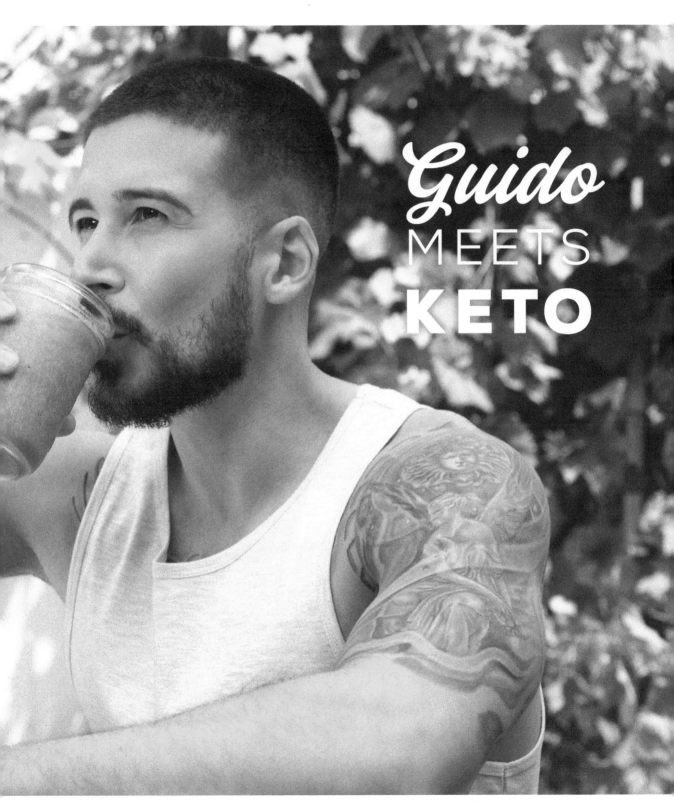

Guido

MEETS

KETO

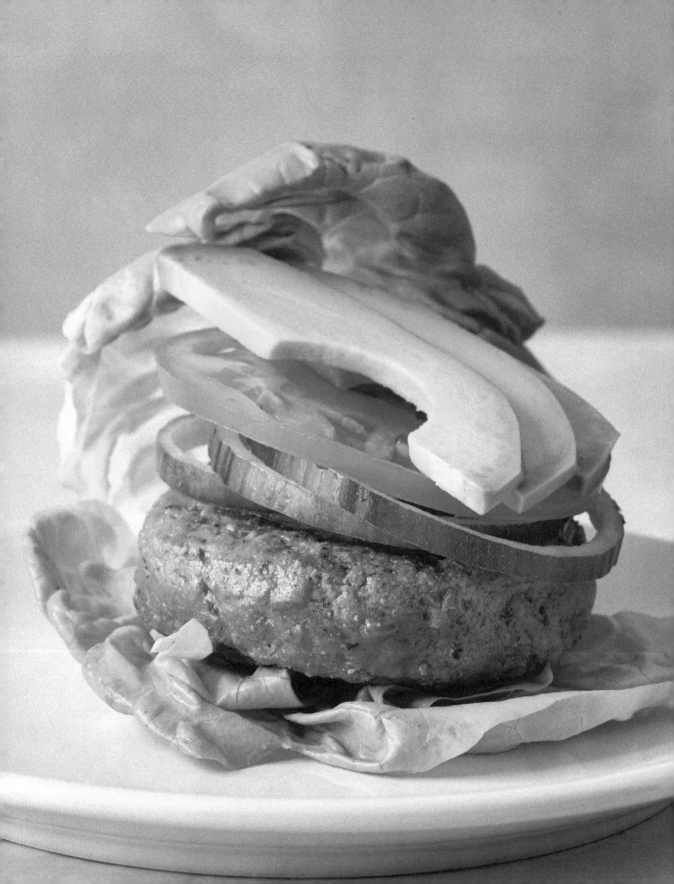

Body by Keto

The Story Behind Keto Guido

It's kind of crazy that I ended up becoming the Keto Guido, because eating keto is definitely not in my DNA. Everyone who watched *Jersey Shore* knows I come from a big, traditional Italian family. Food is everything in Italian culture, and I picked up my eating habits from my family. The reason food is so important to Italians is that it represents home, warmth, generosity, traditions, and love of the family. It's about coming together and celebrating, and you do that over a delicious meal—one that usually revolves around pastas and a pile of bread. Growing up, my family ate a lot of that stuff, and they thought about nutrition differently from how we do today. For instance, they demonized fat, but didn't flinch at eating cereal, sugar, and of course, lots of pasta. So I ate that way and thought it was healthy, too.

To be fair, that's what we all learned in school in the '90s with the food pyramid: Limit your fats, eat lots of grains. We learned that fat is bad and carbs are good. Unfortunately, that led to a lot of us thinking grains are way healthier than they actually are—me included. It finally became clear to me when I learned about keto and started putting it into action. I was amazed at how much better I felt— right away. The bottom line is we need to rethink everything we were taught about nutrition if we want to get healthy.

It's kind of ironic that I'm leaner now than I was back when *Jersey Shore* was first starting because I remember thinking I was probably too small when I applied to be on the show. I'd finished up college and taken the LSAT—like, I was ready to go to law school and become a lawyer. But I'd always wanted to be on camera and my friends knew it, so one of them sent me the *Jersey Shore* application as a joke. I figured they were looking for big, muscular guidos who were all tan with spiky hair, but I filled out the application anyway. I didn't hear anything until a year later when they called me up . . . and the rest is history.

I've tried a bunch of diets over the years, mostly because I've found myself in front of a lot of pasta and a lot of alcohol over the past decade—and with that combo, it's really easy to gain some weight if you let your guard down. My genetics don't allow me to eat whatever I want—if I smell a piece of bread I gain five pounds! So I'd diet to try to drop those pounds, to feel healthier, and even just to try to get more energy so I could keep up with my crazy busy schedule.

I did different diets for years, even some low-carb ones, and they pretty much always went the same way. I would start strong, drop some weight, and then I'd gain it back again. I was yo-yo dieting. Those diets couldn't really stick because they always felt like temporary fixes. I was hungry and unhappy about it most of the time. Plus—I didn't make this public until a few years back—I've had anxiety for my entire life. It's been going on since I was a kid, and I've always tried to take steps to keep it in check. But that means I can't be on a diet that makes me feel worse—I need it to make me feel better. (By the way, I'm not saying keto is going to get rid of anxiety, but when you have anxiety, the last thing you want is to add to it with food that makes you physically feel like crap.) So the crash diets never felt like something I could keep up for six months—or for life. Keto is different. Keto is the only diet I've been able to stick to. I'm now at four years and counting. And I haven't thought of it as a diet in a long time—now it's a way of life.

Why can I stick with keto when I couldn't stick with anything else? Because it works so damn well. Once you start eating keto, your body feels so much better that you don't even want to go back. And that's really what's important when it comes to the way you eat—finding a way to be healthy long-term that feels good and doesn't leave you hungry. (Add on to that how much better you start looking, and you *really* won't want to go back.)

I found out about keto randomly in 2015 when I was listening to Adam Carolla's podcast. He had a fitness expert on there as a guest, Vinnie Tortorich, who started talking about this diet where you could get healthy and lose weight without giving up delicious things like bacon and butter. These days keto's been normalized, so saying that kind of stuff isn't a huge deal. But back then, it seemed crazy to me that it could be a healthy way to eat. But . . . in a funny way, the more I listened to him, the more it made sense to me. I always knew that eating a steak made me feel better than eating a dish of pasta. And eating something buttery never made me feel sick the way too much sugar would. Growing up, I saw my mom try Atkins and lose a bunch of weight. I wrote it off as a fad diet, but I did register that maybe carbs weren't so healthy if cutting them was such a straightforward way to lose weight.

Anyway, after I heard that podcast, I started researching keto as much as I could, listening to other podcasts and buying books on the subject. What I learned was that eating fat *isn't* bad for your body—the thing that's bad is eating simple carbs which cause inflammation and poor gut health. I love cooking, so I bought a keto cookbook, started actually eating this way, and I've never looked back. Keto's definitely changed my life, and I want to help people change theirs, too. Once you've been doing keto for a while and you've experienced how good it makes you feel, you start to look at food differently and—sorry to scare you—you'll start to see how everyone else is poisoning themselves with what they eat.

Ever since I ate just the cheese off my pizza on the first episode of *Jersey Shore Family Vacation*, fans have been coming to me with questions about keto. They see the transformation in my body. They hear me talk about how much better I feel—better than I've ever felt—and they want to feel that way, too. I want to help them (and you!) get started, I want to share everything I've learned along the way, and I want to teach people how to make amazing keto meals that are so good you won't miss grains or sugar at all. I swear it's possible.

It's why I started my Keto Guido Instagram (@ketoguido) and why I've basically become a keto evangelist. And it's why I'm writing this book now. I'm not a nutritionist, I'm just a guy who actually lives this stuff. Keto has been life-changing for me and I want to help people by showing them what I've learned so it can be life-changing for them, too.

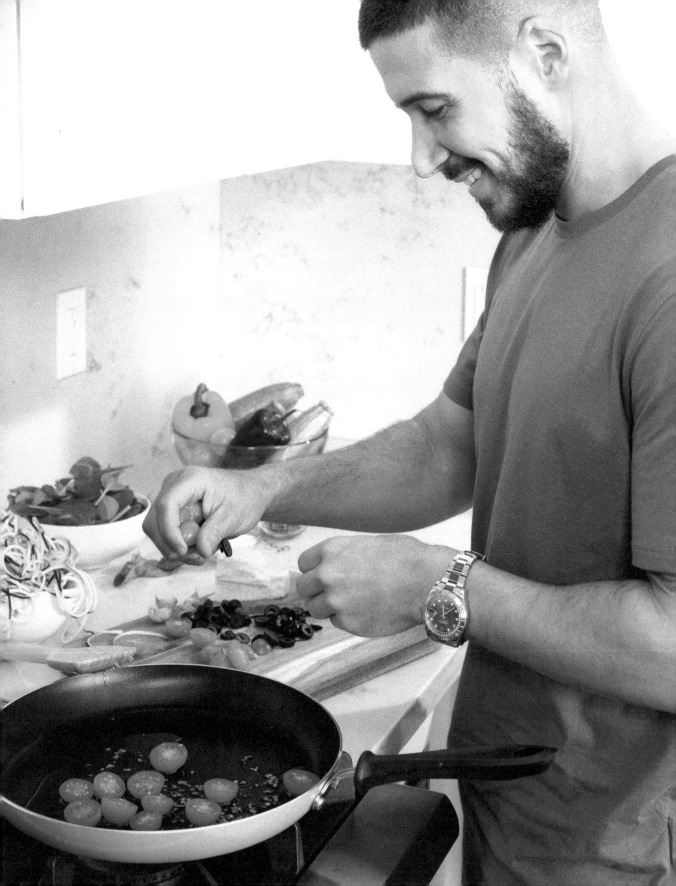

My Take on Keto

I did a ton of research on the keto diet early on to figure out how to get started. (You can check out some of the best books and websites that helped me on page 242.) And look, as I said, I'm not an expert, so for the sake of this book, I worked with health coach Karissa Long, who gets into the science on page 11. But I *am* a guy who's been living keto for several years, and there are some basic concepts and principles that everyone who's thinking about keto should know right up front.

Basic Concepts

The science behind keto is complex, but there are two basic things you need to understand in order to do keto:

- Eat high-fat foods that fill you up and satisfy your taste buds (animal fats, avocado, olive oil, cheese, etc.).
- Ditch all simple carbs and sugars (no bread, pasta, candy, etc.).

Doing these two things gets your body burning fat for energy rather than carbs. This fat-burning state is called "ketosis." And when you break the cycle of relying on carbs for energy, you stop craving them. It's that simple.

Guiding Principles

1. **Renovate your mind.** Keto totally changes how you think about what is and isn't healthy. That's why it's been easy for me to stick to it: Now that I've renovated my mind, I honestly don't even want to go back to putting donuts and Doritos in my mouth again. Of course, I know they taste good, but what they do to my body just isn't worth it.

   The biggest part of retraining your mind is recognizing that pretty much all the "good" carbs you've been eating your whole life aren't so good after all. Like, you probably think of whole wheat bread and oatmeal as healthy, and that things like cupcakes and potato chips aren't. Right? The truth is that while there *is* a difference in those items in terms of nutrients, there's not much difference in terms of how your body ends up processing and using them. Your body handles that cupcake basically the same way it handles the whole wheat bread. Crazy, right? It's true. Basically: All carbs break down into sugar, so ultimately your body processes whole wheat the same way it processes white sugar—it doesn't really distinguish between "good carbs" and "bad carbs"—especially when we are talking about any food that's been processed. Some people will talk about the difference between simple carbs (like the cupcake) and complex carbs (like the whole wheat bread). There is a carb hierarchy, for sure, with some being better than others. That whole wheat bread will take your body longer to digest than the cupcake. But if you think that wheat bread is better than white bread, or that gluten-free pasta is healthier than white pasta—well, that's where people make the biggest mistake because all of those items turn into sugar inside your body.

And that's not all. You wouldn't eat a candy bar for breakfast because it's not healthy, but you probably *would* eat a granola bar. Well . . . they have the same amount of sugar and carbs in them. Some of those granola bars or the yogurt you eat for breakfast can have like 10 sugar cubes in them. Imagine eating 10 sugar cubes by themselves for breakfast! You would feel sick. But because they are hidden in a "healthy" bar we think it's okay. Sure, it's common sense that an apple is better than a candy bar, but if you eat a lot of apples, you're still overdoing it with the sugar. And that's not good if you're trying to lose weight or make your body work more efficiently. Once you get that in your head and make the mental shift, you'll stop feeling like you're missing out by not eating carbs—and you'll start feeling *grateful* you're not eating them because you realize they were keeping you from feeling good, from losing weight, and getting healthier. So from now on, let's look at processed bread like it's cake, orange juice like it's soda, and granola bars like they're candy bars.

2. **Aim to Eat in Macro Percentages.** Macros are the three basic parts of all your food: fat, protein, and carbohydrates. With keto, you want to balance your macros so you're eating mostly fat, some protein, and very, very few carbs. The percentages to aim for are 75% fat, 20% protein, 5% carbs. The goal is for your macros to wind up around there every day, (but not necessarily every meal), which does give you a little more freedom.

Figuring out macros might sound complicated at first, but they become second nature pretty quick. Macros are one of my favorite parts of keto because they keep things simple. So rather than counting calories, I decide what I'm going to eat in relation to the other things I eat. Like, I love eating bacon. And on keto, you can eat it. Not turkey bacon, not bacon where you soak up the grease with a paper towel—real, straight-up bacon. Bacon's got a lot of fat, but not a ton of protein, so I know if I'm eating it at one meal, maybe I'll have a salmon salad at the next meal to balance out my macros.

You may be wondering how calories fit into all of this. If you're trying to lose weight I suggest consuming less calories than you are burning and having smaller portions. But here's the funny thing—on keto, you usually end up eating fewer calories naturally because the food is so satisfying. At this point, I'm pretty sure I burn more than I eat without thinking about it. That's the beauty of keto. You can end up having a caloric deficit easily without even consciously counting calories, especially if you pair it with exercise and intermittent fasting (which I'll talk about later).

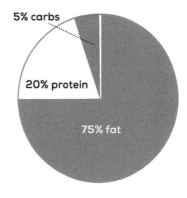

3. **Eat Whole Foods. Avoid Processed Foods.** Your goal on keto is to eat as many real, whole foods as possible. You've got to avoid processed foods, especially ones with added sugars. Processed foods are, basically, everything you find in the middle of the grocery store, foods that don't exist in nature— like, you can't pick Cheetos off a Cheetos tree. So any foods with added sugar, high-fructose corn syrup, preservatives, and God knows what else— those are processed and you want to avoid them. Those foods are more chemicals than, well, actual food. That's the stuff that's killing us.

Now, when you're eating keto, you're going to wind up buying *some* foods that aren't just meat straight off a cow or vegetables you grew and picked yourself. Anytime you have to buy something that comes packaged, make sure you read the ingredients on the package carefully. If you stick to foods that have very short lists of ingredients—and you recognize what all of the ingredients are—your body is going to thank you.

Why Keto Succeeds Where Other Diets Fail

Dieting is frigging terrible. I know that because I've spent so much time doing it. And the reason so many diets fail: They're not satisfying. You're either always hungry or you feel deprived (and maybe proud of yourself for succeeding at being deprived). That's not the way Mother Nature intended for us to live and eat. Keto is different. You're eating foods that are rich, satisfying, and taste good. (Seriously, if you've been eating low-fat cheese and avoiding dark meat to be "healthy" all these years, keto's going to blow your mind.) With keto, you don't feel like you're constantly hungry or depriving yourself of the good stuff because your body is finally running the way it evolved to run. That's why keto sticks when other diets don't.

Keto Diet 101

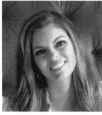

by Karissa Long

Global health coach, CEO/founder of Clean Keto Lifestyle, and author of the ketogenic lifestyle and cookbook Clean Keto Lifestyle

As a global health coach, ketogenic expert, and graduate of the Institute for Integrative Nutrition, I have been living the keto life and helping others live it, too, for almost a decade with my company, Clean Keto Lifestyle, LLC, which provides keto coaching programs, courses, and meal plans.

I discovered the ketogenic diet during my struggle with a debilitating autoimmune disease. Through extensive scientific research, reviewing thousands of medical studies, and using myself as a guinea pig, I was able to master the keto diet and put my autoimmune disease into remission.

But that wasn't the only incredible result I experienced with the keto diet. I also shed excess weight, cleared my acne, improved my sleep, and boosted my energy. It was then that I realized how powerful the ketogenic diet truly is. Keto isn't a fad, it isn't a quick fix, rather it is the way our bodies were designed to operate.

The Body's Two Fuel Sources

The goal of the ketogenic diet is simple: to transition your body from using glucose as fuel to using ketones as fuel. Most people don't realize this, but your body has two fuel sources. Let's break down each one.

The first one is **glucose**. Glucose is produced by your body from the carbohydrates you eat, such as grains, breads, pastas, sugar, and starches. Glucose is easily produced by the body to use for energy, but it is not long-lasting, causes blood sugar spikes, and when you don't burn all of the glucose that your body produces, it is stored as **fat** in the form of triglycerides. I repeat, your body stores the excess glucose in your fat cells. And this goes for *all carbs*. You may have heard the term **glycemic index**, which measures how quickly food raises your blood sugar using a ranking system of 0 to 100, with pure sugar having a value of 100. Simple carbs that are fast burning are high on the GI scale, while complex carbs that are slow burning are lower on the glycemic index. While complex carbs do keep your blood sugar more level over time, at the end of the day, *all carbs still turn into glucose*, and whatever excess that is not burned as energy by the body will be stored as fat.

The other fuel source is **ketones**. Ketones are produced in your liver from stored fat. Yes, you heard me correctly: You can turn stored fat cells into energy. Ketones are a long-lasting fuel that provide consistent energy with no afternoon crashes. When you use ketones for energy, your body is using its own stored fat as fuel, thus you start shedding weight.

The goal of the ketogenic diet is for your body to start burning ketones for energy instead of glucose. When the body takes stored fat through the liver and produces ketones (small molecules used as fuel throughout the body), it is called **ketosis**.

How do you get into ketosis? It is all about what you eat and the ratio of the macronutrients (also known as "macros") that you consume. There are three types of macronutrients: fats, proteins, and carbohydrates. On the ketogenic diet, your daily macronutrient breakdown should be as follows:

- 75% fat
- 20% protein
- 5% carbohydrates

At first, 75% fat might sound excessive, but consuming healthy fats is the key to keto. Fat is actually the most essential macronutrient the body needs. It also keeps you feeling full and satisfied, it keeps cravings away, and it is 100 percent necessary for you to get into ketosis. And the best part? There are plenty of healthy fats to choose from: extra-virgin olive oil, avocados, nuts, seeds, coconut oil, ghee, butter, cheese, and cream, all in addition to animal fats. So embrace fats!

So What Is the Keto Diet?

In the most basic terms, the keto diet is a low-carb, moderate-protein, high-fat diet designed to exhaust sugar levels in your body and prompt it to instead use fat as a source of energy.

Keto Versus

Paleo: While keto does have some similarities to the Paleo diet (i.e., grains, legumes, and refined sugars are off-limits), there are a few differences, as well. The main difference is macro-guidance. The ketogenic diet has specific macronutrient guidelines that are to be followed in order to get your body into ketosis (the primary goal). The Paleo diet provides no macronutrient guidelines, and its primary goal is to return you to a way of eating that mirrors what humans ate in the Paleolithic era. Other differences relate to the types of foods consumed on each diet. Paleo allows participants to consume unlimited fruit, natural sweeteners (think honey and maple syrup), and starchy veggies, which are consumed sparingly if at all on keto. Keto, on the other hand, allows for dairy consumption, which is avoided on Paleo.

Atkins: Dr. Robert Atkins became popular in the 1970s when he promoted a low-carb diet that focused primarily on restricting your carbohydrate intake to 100 grams or fewer. Unlike the ketogenic diet, the Atkins diet set no specific guidelines on fat and protein intake. As a result, Americans began eating mounds of chicken wings, steak, and bacon to their heart's desire with no concern for protein and fat levels. The ketogenic diet upgrades Atkins by focusing on specific fat and protein levels to ensure you reap the benefits of being in ketosis.

How Genetics Factor In

Like everything in life, genetics do play a role in the ketogenic diet and your results. Each person converts and burns carbs at a different rate since genes are involved in energy metabolism. So how your body reacts to varying kinds and amounts of carbohydrates can be very different from another person. Someone with a faster metabolism can generally eat more carbs than one with a slower metabolism.

While the ketogenic diet and recommended macronutrient ratios work for most people, it is not the be-all and end-all for every single person. Some adjustments have to be made to fit *your* body, because your unique genetics play a huge role. These adjustments could be experimenting with the number of grams of carbs consumed, or potentially removing dairy from your diet, or even eating more protein each day. Pay attention to how you are feeling and how your body is reacting to the diet. In general, the keto diet works well for most people because your body is wired to be burning ketones as fuel, plus you are ridding your body of inflammatory sugars and grains, as well as embracing nourishing and healing high-quality fats.

Keto Diet Myths Debunked

There is a ton of misinformation related to the ketogenic diet. Let's take a look at some of the common misunderstandings.

Myth 1: The keto diet is unhealthy and low in fiber.
Answer: The keto diet is actually full of essential amino acids, vitamins, and minerals. It is also very high in fiber when followed correctly by focusing on whole foods. The cornerstones of the ketogenic diet are healthy fats, quality protein, and organic vegetables, so you will actually be upgrading your nutrition.

Myth 2: Glucose is the preferred fuel for the brain.

Answer: Your brain has something called a "blood barrier," which is a very tight barrier that only allows certain components of your blood to penetrate it. Glucose is actually one component that can't seamlessly cross the blood brain barrier, which can result in inconsistent energy to the brain. Ketones, however, are small enough to cross this blood brain barrier and can facilitate a constant supply of energy to the brain. That means no more brain fog or 3 p.m. afternoon crash! Besides that, ketones provide more energy per unit (in oxygen) than glucose, meaning ketones are actually a more efficient fuel source.

Myth 3: The keto diet will increase my cholesterol.

Answer: This is actually a half myth. While doing the ketogenic diet, your levels of LDL cholesterol (the bad one) goes down, while the good cholesterol known as HDL goes up. This improved ratio helps protect your health.

I know from working with Vinny that he believes what's more important than your cholesterol numbers is having clear, healthy arteries, which is much more a function of reducing chronic inflammation in your body than focusing on cholesterol levels. Chronic inflammation is created in the body from a diet of processed foods, sugar, refined oils, and artificial ingredients and can lead to hardening of the arteries and increased risk for heart attacks. With a ketogenic diet, inflammatory sugar and refined grains are already removed from your diet, and when you layer in quality fats, proteins, and vegetables, you are well on your way to keeping chronic inflammation at bay and having healthier arteries, which is what people are usually concerned with when they ask about cholesterol levels.

Keto Benefits

Let's review the numerous benefits of the ketogenic diet in detail.

1. **Weight Loss.** By definition, being in a state of ketosis means you are burning stored fat for energy. Weight loss happens quickly and can be significant because you are turning your body into a fat-burning machine when you are producing ketones. It's simply body science.

2. **Increased Energy.** As I described earlier, ketones are able to cross the brain's blood barrier to provide consistent and superior energy, which means your energy levels will skyrocket in comparison to using glucose for fuel. Once again, this phenomenon is a result of your body operating off a more efficient fuel source in the form of ketones.

3. **Reduced Inflammation.** Chronic inflammation is the root cause of many serious health conditions. A huge benefit of being in ketosis is that it can lower inflammation because free radical production (which is extremely inflammatory) is reduced when you begin burning ketones for energy instead of glucose. Also, when you remove sugar and refined carbohydrates from your diet, as you do with keto, you consequently eliminate many inflammation-producing additives, artificial ingredients, preservatives, and sweeteners. Less inflammation in the body leads to a multitude of other benefits, including better sleep, less acne, improved skin condition, better muscle tone, and a balanced mood.

4. **Relief from and reversal of symptoms of some autoimmune conditions.** Your digestive system and gut microbiome play a huge part in your immune system and in autoimmune disease. The ketogenic diet promotes the healing of your gut lining because you are ridding your body of the foods that can cause holes in your gut. This healing combined with consistently reduced inflammation can make it an effective tool for reversing the symptoms of autoimmune conditions.

My List of What to Choose and What to Lose

Foods to Eat

- Berries: blackberries, blueberries, raspberries, strawberries
- Cacao and sugar-free chocolate
- Cruciferous vegetables: arugula, bok choy, broccoli, Brussels sprouts, cabbage, cauliflower, collard greens, kale
- Drinks: coffee, sparkling water, unsweetened tea, water
- Extra-virgin olive oil, avocado oil, coconut oil
- Fatty fruit: avocado, olives
- Flour: almond flour, almond meal, coconut flour
- Full-fat coconut milk and cream
- Full-fat dairy: cheese, heavy whipping cream, organic cream cheese, sour cream
- Grass-fed butter and/or ghee
- Grass-fed meats: beef and lamb
- Herbs and dried spices: basil, oregano, pepper, rosemary, thyme
- Nuts: almonds, macadamia nuts, pecans, walnuts
- Other vegetables: asparagus, celery, cucumbers, onions, peppers, summer squash, tomatoes, zucchini
- Pasture-raised chicken and pork
- Pasture-raised eggs
- Pink Himalayan salt
- Seeds: chia seeds, flax seeds, sunflower seeds
- Sweetener: erythritol, monk fruit, stevia, xylitol
- Uncured bacon (no sugar added)
- Wild-caught seafood

Foods to Avoid

- Dried fruit
- Factory-farmed fish
- Flour: all-purpose flour, corn flour, rice flour, wheat flour
- Fruits other than berries: apples, bananas (for the most part), dates, mangos, oranges, etc.
- Grains: bread, cereal, farro, rice, pasta
- Higher carb nuts: cashews, pistachios
- Legumes: beans, chickpeas, peanuts
- Low-quality oils: canola, corn, safflower, soybean, sunflower, vegetable
- Margarine
- Milk
- Processed meats: canned meats, cold cuts with chemical preservatives, conventional hot dogs, etc.
- Starchy vegetables: beets, butternut squash, corn, potatoes, yams
- Sugary drinks: energy drinks, fruit juice, soda
- Sugary sweeteners: agave, maple syrup, sugar

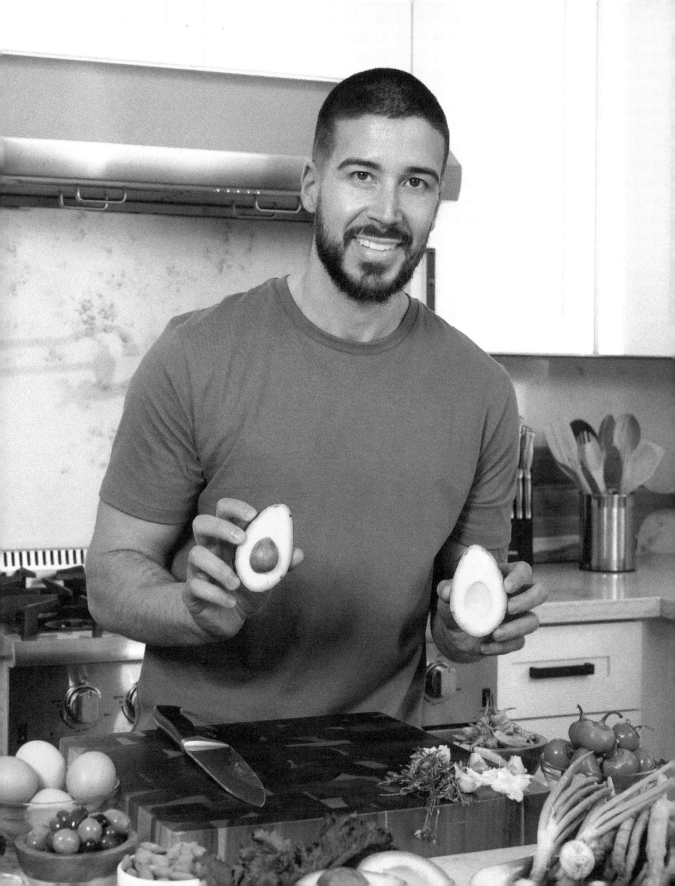

How I Eat

I've been eating keto for so long at this point, I don't have to think too hard about it, which is a beautiful thing. It's one of the reasons I love this diet—it's not *really a diet*, it's a way of eating, and it's easy. It's about listening to my body and giving it what it wants. It definitely doesn't want simple carbs, like most grains or sugars. My body usually doesn't want too much dairy, either. I also do intermittent fasting, which means that sometimes my body wants to eat two meals a day, sometimes three, sometimes just one. Basically, I don't force myself to eat if I'm not hungry, and honestly, I don't get crazy hungry the way I used to. You'll get to this good place with keto, too, but when you're just starting out, you're going to want to pay closer attention to get on the right track. That means you'll want to count macros, figure out what knocks you out of ketosis, and plan out your meals in advance. (Check out the one-week meal plan on page 34 which will help you get a jump on all of that.)

No Grains

My meals are high in fat and tend to align with keto guidelines pretty well, but I don't always stick to them 100 percent. Some of the stuff I eat is more "Paleo" than "keto"—like I'll have a little honey or an apple once in a while or a grain-free tortilla. But one thing I'm not very flexible on is grains. Even before I was aware of keto, I knew I felt better after I ate protein than after I ate grains. And now that my body is off grains, when I do have them, I don't feel great. That bad feeling is a good thing, by the way. My body *should* reject it—it's like my body is saying "this stuff is poison."

Keep Dairy in Check

One of the big things that draws people to keto is dairy. "I can eat all the cheese I want? Hell yeah, I'm in, sign me up." And it's sort of true. Dairy products are high in fat, they fill you up, keep you satiated. Plus dairy tastes really good. But for me, I like to keep my dairy in check. It goes back to listening to your body. I listened to mine, and I found it didn't feel as good or run as efficiently when I was packing in lots of dairy. (For me, it can cause some inflammation.) So now I use dairy more like a tool rather than an "every meal, every day" kind of thing. I'll throw a little cheese into my eggs to punch up the flavor, but I'm not eating eggs with a huge brick of Cheddar on the side every morning. And when I do use dairy, I always go full-fat. The more it tastes like cow, the better.

Clean, Not Lean

When someone finds out I eat keto, they usually say something like, "So what, you just eat bacon and butter all day?" Technically, yeah, that could be considered keto, but it's what I like to call "dirty keto," and it's not how I eat. Keto isn't about shoving as much meat and cheese in your body as you can fit, it's about making your body healthier by eating the foods it really wants and needs. That's why I stick to more of a "clean keto" diet. That means I eat animal fats and dairy, but I also balance them out with lots of vegetables. I don't eat an entire plate of bacon, I eat a few strips of bacon. And if I want a snack, I won't just hit a convenience store and buy up all their Slim Jims, I'll have some nuts or vegetables or a hardboiled egg. Some people ask me how it's "clean" if I'm eating animal fats. Think of it this way: If you're eating an animal from nose to tail, you're gonna run into fat somewhere. It's natural, it's clean, and it's how our ancestors ate.

Sweeteners

Just because you go keto doesn't mean you can never eat anything sweet again. There are sweeteners that are keto-friendly, things like monk fruit extract, stevia, erythritol, xylitol, and allulose. I'll use them in my recipes the way I use dairy—to punch up the flavor of something. But I don't use them that much because my goal is to put whole foods in my body, and artificial sweeteners are not whole foods. So if you do want to sweeten something, you can, but don't go overboard. Experiment, and use the sweetener that agrees with you best. I like to use monk fruit extract, which is more natural than the others.

Honestly, sometimes if I want something sweet, I'll use a sweetener like coconut sugar or organic honey. Those kinds of sugars aren't allowed on keto normally, but they're natural to the Earth, and they're fine on Paleo, so I'm okay with eating them in small amounts. For the desserts in this book, I use monk fruit extract in case you want to stay more "pure keto" than me, but if you want to swap the monk

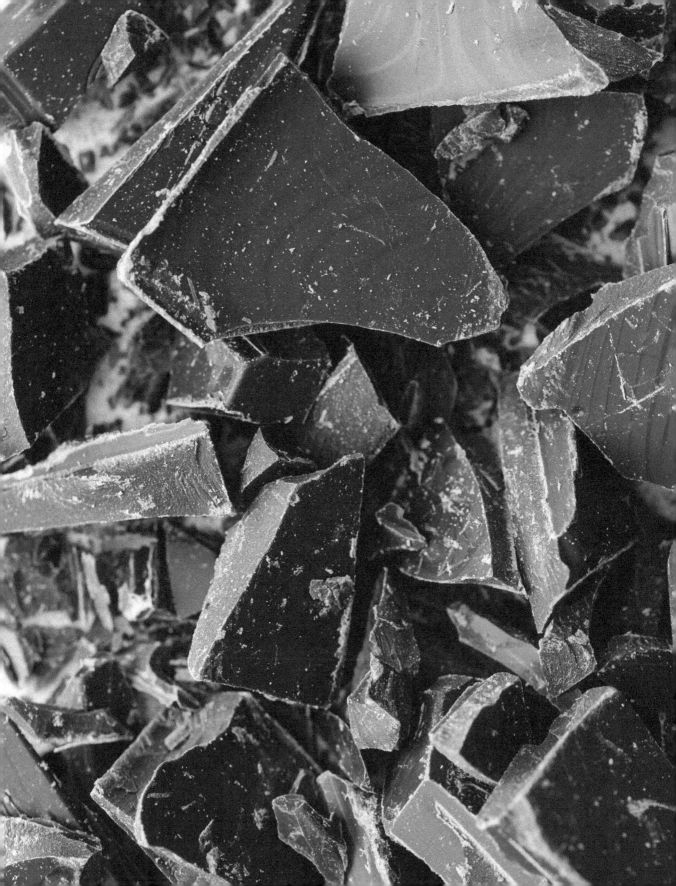

fruit for honey or coconut sugar, I give you permission. Just make sure it's only once in a while so you don't mess up your ketosis.

Cheating

Sometimes you're in a situation where you decide to cheat and have a small amount of simple carbs. Like when I'm filming *Jersey Shore*, drinking is my cheat since there are simple carbs in alcohol. When I need to drink for a club appearance or on the show, I'll try to stick to a lower-carb alcohol, like liquor or some red wines. But one thing I never have is any kind of sugary soda or juice.

Cheating isn't great to do, but at the end of the day, remember that keto is a lifestyle, not some fad diet that you have to stress out about. So if you need a little something extra here and there to stay keto the rest of the time, that's okay.

Now that I've been on keto for a while, for example, I can eat regular, non-keto pizza occasionally. Don't get me wrong—it will set me back and it will *for sure* take me out of ketosis (and I might not feel very good after), but I can afford to do it every once in a while because I've built a solid foundation the rest of the time. Basically, I want you to understand that keto is not a prison sentence. If the idea of never being able to eat regular birthday cake on your birthday again bums you out, it's okay to make that exception. The aim of the Keto Guido diet is to get it right most of the time, and then treat yourself every once in a while if you need to. If knowing you have a cheat meal coming up motivates you to keep going with keto, use that as a tool.

While you want to stay away from grains in general, I personally believe that you can eat a small amount of grains or something else starchy every once in a while just to make sure your body doesn't forget how to handle them. You want to be able to digest anything, even if it's not something you eat regularly anymore. So a healthier way I sometimes cheat is that I'll have a low-carb Paleo wrap on occasion. It's not technically keto, but it still fits my policy of being low carb, and it helps keep me metabolically flexible without being really bad for me.

Snacks

Snacking isn't a huge part of keto. The high-fat foods you eat do such a good job of filling you up that you won't need many snacks. And when you're on keto, you're eating like our ancestors ate: They didn't worry about snacks, they just ate when they were hungry and they had food available. That said, we're not cavemen sitting around sharing a mastodon. In these modern times, sometimes you need a snack to tide you over until your next meal. I know I do sometimes when I'm traveling a lot or on the road for work, or even between takes of filming *Jersey Shore*.

My go-to is uncured beef jerky (from a keto-approved brand that I know has no sugar added), or maybe a handful of macadamia nuts, or a protein shake. I also make great homemade energy bars. They're maybe a little more Paleo than keto, but they're still a really good snack option. I use things like grass-fed butter, cayenne, sea salt, honey, tahini, maca, and turmeric.

Macro Counting

When you're starting out and just learning about keto, it's good to count macros to make sure your body gets adjusted. But after a while you won't need to do it anymore. Honestly, I don't count macros anymore. When I did other diets, I hated counting calories, and a big reason I do keto is because it's the opposite of counting calories. Here's how I look at it: Once your body is in ketosis and it's used to fueling itself off the right things, it will start naturally running that way. There's actually a term for it: fat-adapted. That means your body is used to running off ketones, so even if you have some sugar or simple carbs once in a while, your body won't immediately go back to running on glucose. (Check out Karissa's breakdown of the science on page 11.) And guess what? It doesn't take your body that long to get fat-adapted. For most people, it's only about four weeks. Being fat-adapted helps you have longer sustainable energy so you eat less. (Unlike when you're running off glucose and have to get your energy source with every quick hit of sugar.)

So no, I don't count macros anymore. And once you've kickstarted keto and you're really rolling, you won't need to count them, either. The bottom line is that on the Keto Guido diet, once your body has adapted, your macros don't have to be so strict. It's a simple way of life: Eat good fats, some protein, and veggies. If I need to lose weight, body fat, or really hit a goal because of my line of work, then I can fine-tune it by using apps or tools like fitness bands. So I use that stuff to get on track, but ultimately this way of life doesn't require that year-round, which is what I love about it.

My Tips for Getting the Most Out of Keto

Don't be overwhelmed by counting macros. They're helpful at first, but eventually you won't need to obsess over them. You should enjoy your life and not always be sitting around counting macros. And if you aren't perfectly at 75% fat, 20% protein, 5% carbs every day, don't worry. If you just get close, think of how much *better* that is compared to how you used to eat. Do I always have the perfect ratio, and am I always in ketosis? The answer is no. Because I don't always have to be in order to lose weight, and neither do you. This lifestyle as a whole keeps you healthy and eating fewer calories naturally. So my advice is to stick pretty close to it, but also give yourself a break and take the pressure off.

Plan ahead. Know what you're going to eat for the day so you can avoid big hunger swings and avoid finding yourself in a situation where you don't have keto food available.

Vary it up. Eat different foods every day. That way you won't get bored, and you'll be getting different nutrients and benefits from different things.

Listen to your body. The basics of keto are the same for everyone, but when it comes to the little things, listen to your body. As I said before, I don't do well with lots of dairy, but maybe you do. Try different keto foods and see how you feel. No one's forcing you to eat bacon-wrapped steaks cooked in butter if you don't like them.

Make it sustainable. If there's a food you really love that's natural but not keto, it's okay to have a little every once in a while. For example, I sometimes use a little bit of banana, fresh-squeezed orange juice, or honey when I'm cooking. Having them in small portions works well for me and keeps me going. Is it cheating? Sure, but if that's what makes you stick to this way of eating most of the time, it's probably worth it.

Work out. Working out isn't technically a part of keto, but you'll get the best results if you have a regular exercise routine.

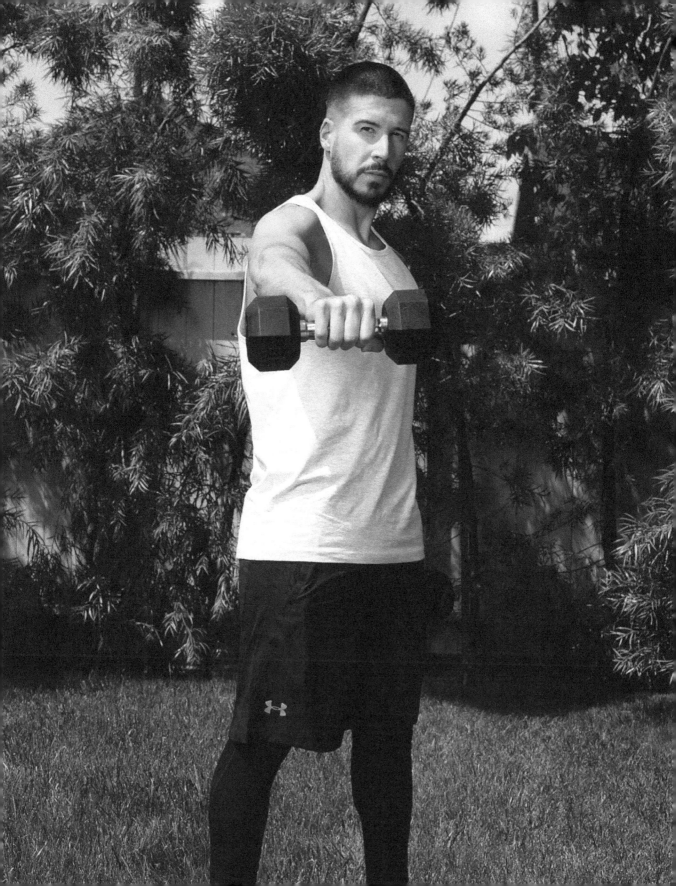

The G of GTL (Gym, Tan & Laundry)

Eating keto naturally makes me feel good, but working out makes me feel even better. I work out pretty much every day. I usually work out in the morning before I eat anything. Because I do intermittent fasting and my body is fueling itself off fat, I have plenty of energy. Then I'll eat something when I get home, maybe a shake or some eggs or another protein. I mix up my workouts, from cardio to weight lifting to boxing, and I'll even do two workouts a day when I have the time. Keto probably isn't the best way to get huge—those guys are eating a ton of protein and also lots of strategic carbs—but when you put keto together with regular exercise, it's a hell of a way to get fit and healthy at the same time. Remember that no matter what you're eating, you still want to burn calories. Pairing keto with working out helps you naturally be in a caloric deficit, which makes losing weight and staying strong easier.

I Did It and So Can You

I jumped into keto basically on a hunch, and it completely transformed my life. It can do that for you, too. Even if you've tried a bunch of diets and failed, keto can change your life because it's *so* different than any other diet. The food is amazing, I'm literally never hungry, I can stick to the diet at any restaurant or in any situation, and it changed my way of thinking so that I don't even *miss* all the simple carbs and sugars I used to eat. I feel healthier than I ever have before, and I look the best I've ever looked, too. Keto changed my life, and I know it can change yours, too. And even if it sounds hard, trust me, it's worth it. You got this.

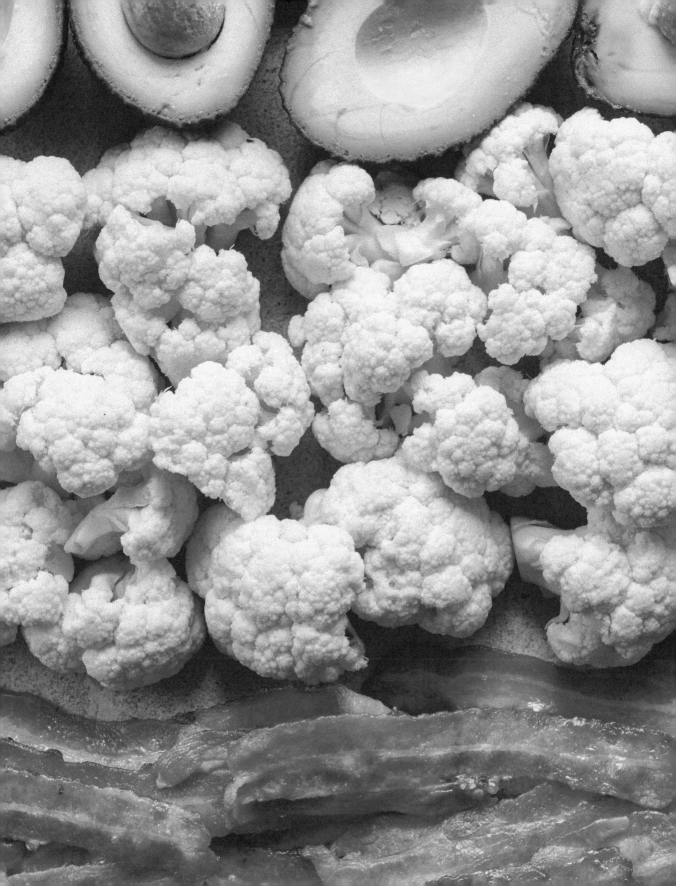

2

My Keto Kitchen

When you're cleaning out your kitchen and restocking it with brand-new foods, remember the principles behind keto: high fat, moderate protein, low carb. And most importantly: REAL, WHOLE FOODS. I'm putting it in all caps so you see it loud and clear. That's going to influence what you add to your kitchen—and what you toss. Personally, I like to eat the Mediterranean-inspired diet I grew up with as part of a Sicilian family, so you'll see how that influences the ingredients I recommend here and also the recipes later in the book.

Before You Do Anything

Before we jump into buying a bunch of ingredients, I want to slow things down for a minute. You've obviously got a reason for wanting to do keto, and I want to make sure you stay focused on that reason so you can do the most effective version of keto for you. I'm also going to steer you toward staples and simple meals that use common ingredients, so you'll have lots of good leftovers. Let's keep it easy.

Get Clear on Your Goals

What's your motivation for doing keto? Do you want to lose weight? Maintain your weight? Get healthier overall? Are you fighting an autoimmune disorder? Keto works for all of those, but the approach can be a little different in each case. For example, if you're trying to lose weight, you'll want smaller portions. Keep your goals in mind as you go through this chapter and through the recipes later to find what works best for what you want to achieve—and for your taste buds. Because if you like the food *and* the results, it's going to make keto even easier to stick with. Find the ingredients you're most likely to use and enjoy cooking with. Cooking and eating on keto shouldn't feel like a chore.

Make the Easy Stuff

I hope one day you're making crazy complicated keto recipes that belong in five-star restaurants. One day. But for now, we're going to keep it simple. Let's focus on meals that are easy to pull off and enjoy, and make for a lot of leftovers for those lazy days when you don't feel like cooking.

On your first day for breakfast, try cooking an egg in butter and eating it with a side of bacon (page 50). If you're feeling ambitious, maybe also make a handful of sautéed spinach. One of the easiest lunches I throw together is a bowl with tuna mixed with avocado mayo and some chopped avocado (page 99). This stuff is all super quick and simple to make, and you can always vary it up by substituting in other staples. Eventually, you'll get more ambitious with what you make. For now, keep it basic.

Enjoy the Leftovers

If you feel like you've got to spend an hour in the kitchen preparing every meal for keto, that's not gonna last. That's where leftovers come in. Always try to make multiple portions when you're cooking, and make stuff that keeps well in the fridge. My recipes are geared toward leaving you with lots of leftovers you can eat throughout the week when you don't have time (or just don't want) to cook.

Also, think about repurposing your leftovers so you don't get bored. If you make chicken thighs for dinner, you could quickly turn the leftovers into chicken salad the next day for a totally different meal that takes a fraction of the prep time of making it from scratch.

Stock Your Kitchen

Having a well-stocked kitchen makes it so much easier to do all the keto cooking you need. And it helps keep you from accidental slip-ups, which is key.

Pantry Foods

Almond flour. Obviously I'm not eating grains on keto, so almond flour is my go-to when I'm making anything that would normally use wheat flour.

Avocado oil. Everyone knows about olive oil, and I've got that for sure, but don't forget about avocado oil. It's one of the healthiest oils. It's got lots of fat and it's great for when I'm cooking something on a high heat (since different oils have different smoke points—see the sidebar on page 30).

Dark chocolate. I've always had a sweet tooth, so if I need to take care of that, a couple squares of dark chocolate gets it done. I try to go with the keto-friendly dark chocolates, which are the ones with the highest amounts of cacao (like 85 percent or higher) and the least sugar.

Everything but the Bagel seasoning. One of the best ways to avoid getting bored with keto food is to vary up your spices and seasonings. Trader Joe's Everything but the Bagel is great, especially on hardboiled eggs or avocado. It takes them from kinda boring to delicious.

Sea salt and pink Himalayan salt. It helps to take in some extra sodium on keto, especially when you're starting out and your body is flushing sodium like crazy. So don't worry about adding salt to what you're eating.

Countertop Foods

Almonds. If you're ever really hungry and need something quick, a handful of almonds should fill you up. Other good nuts are pecans, brazil nuts, macadamia nuts, walnuts, and hazelnuts.

Avocados. Avocados are everywhere in keto. They've got lots of fat and fiber, plus a little avocado makes everything taste better.

Limes. Limes are great for adding flavor to food, or even your water, instead of using something sugary.

Onions. They've got a few carbs, but the flavor they add is totally worth it.

Tomatoes. Same deal as onions. Tomatoes have a few more carbs than a lot of the green vegetables, but I can't cook without 'em. Maybe it's my Italian roots.

Refrigerated Foods

Arugula. It's my favorite green vegetable, so I use it for basically all my salads. I can go through a whole giant container of arugula in just a couple days.

Eggs. I go free-range, cage-free, and pasteurized with my eggs. I like the brown ones, but that's just personal preference.

Grass-fed butter. Always cook with butter, not margarine or Smart Balance. I'd rather cook from a natural product than have a bunch of chemicals.

Olives. Even though I don't eat pasta, I still use a lot of Italian staples. For instance, I *need* to have good olives at all times.

Organic veggies. I buy 'em frozen a lot of the time because I don't always have time to chop my own broccoli. Frozen veggies have the same nutrients as fresh ones, so this is a great time-saver.

Sugar-free, uncured bacon. I don't go crazy and eat a whole package of bacon in one sitting. I'll just have a few slices with my eggs to get my bacon fix. Always check the ingredients list to make sure it doesn't have sugar added.

Know Your Smoke Points

You'll be doing a lot of cooking with ghee, butter, and olive oil on keto. (Ghee is clarified butter, which is butter that's been cooked and strained to get rid of water and milk.)

Something I learned about when I started researching keto was smoke points. A smoke point is the temperature when an oil/fat is so hot that it starts to burn. The smoke point of ghee is around 485°F, the smoke point of butter is 350°F, and the smoke point of olive oil is 405°F.

Those smoke points matter because that's when oil goes from "good" to "bad." At the smoke point, the oil breaks down and turns unhealthy. (That happens at just 225°F for canola oil, by the way, which is an oil you'll find in a lot of processed foods.)

So if you're broiling, deep frying, or stir frying something, ghee is a good choice because of its super-high smoke point. If you're searing, sautéing, or baking things, butter and olive oil are great.

Gather Your Tools

You've probably got the basics in your kitchen already, like frying pans, cutting boards, and knives. If you don't, seriously, go get some knives. How are you cooking anything without knives? Anyway, here are some of the other tools I use all the time that help me make all my different meals.

Outdoor grill. When it's nice out, I grill meat outside all the time. Food off the grill always tastes better, you know? There's something primitive and natural about it. (But if you don't have access to an outdoor grill, you can easily grill things on a **grill pan** on your oven's stovetop.)

Cast iron skillet. I live on Staten Island, and there are some really cold months there. That's when I cook meat inside with my cast iron skillet. It's worth investing in one because they last forever. I swear, you could pass it down to your grandkids. And one important thing to know about using cast iron that my mom taught me is to never wash it with soap!

Slow cooker. I've started using a slow cooker lately, and now I can't go back to life without it. If you're busy like I am, the slow cooker is great because you throw in some stuff before you leave in the morning and it's ready when you get home at night.

Blender. I drink a lot of protein shakes, so I basically can't survive without a blender.

Food processor. A food processor helps make keto meal prep so much faster. If you ever try making cauliflower rice by hand, you'll be buying a food processor the next day.

Thermometer. Since you'll be eating meat, a thermometer is a nice thing to have on hand to make sure you're cooking your meat to the right temperatures. This can mean the difference between a rare steak and a well-done one. Anyone who knows me knows I take my steak temperature *very* seriously. I fight with Pauly D all the time about this because he wants his steak medium-well and I like mine rare. The rare meat is where all the flavor is! I'm half-joking though—to each their own.

Air fryer. While it's not necessary for keto meals, I love using my air fryer to get that crispiness I crave. I use it for all kinds of things—chicken wings, chips, Brussels sprouts, you name it. You'll see that no recipes in this book require an air fryer, but I've given suggestions at the end of some of them for how you can use an air fryer to make the recipe even better.

Toss It

Here are five things you'll want to get out of your kitchen forever because they're secretly really bad for you.

Agave syrup. You may have bought agave syrup to use as a sweetener because it's natural and you heard it's healthier than refined sugar. That's all technically true, but it's still not keto. It's actually way sweeter than refined sugar and it's 90 percent fructose, which means it'll mess with your metabolism. So skip it, unless you've decided that this is your "cheat" sweetener. And even then, only use it once in a while and in small amounts.

Cashews. Not all nuts are good on keto. One ounce of cashews has over 8 grams of carbs, so choose other nuts instead.

Dressing. People overlook dressing because it's just a topping. Well, it's a topping that's often filled with sugar, unhealthy oils, and chemicals that you're pouring on top of your healthy vegetables. That's why I use olive oil, black pepper, and black truffle sea salt on my salads—it's way healthier, and it tastes even better than processed dressing. Change the way you think about dressing—start looking at it like it's maple syrup. It's similar to the way you're changing how you think about a "healthy" granola bar.

Ketchup. Most people don't realize ketchup is loaded up with sugar and, even worse, corn syrup. One tablespoon of regular Heinz ketchup—*1 tablespoon*—has 4 grams of sugar. I personally use Primal Kitchen ketchup, which has much less sugar.

Spice mixes. Spices and seasonings are really important on keto, but check the labels. There are hidden sugars everywhere, so be aware, especially of any spice blends where there is the potential that someone slipped extra stuff in there.

Make it Work for You

The bottom line is you've got to make keto work *for you* if you're going to be able to stick with it. And eventually you'll get into the zone where you'll be able to tweak things to fit you perfectly. Now I can plan out my meals and I know they're keto without even tracking anything. But when I was just starting out, I made a ton of mistakes. It's hard not to. That's why when you're beginning, it can be helpful to have someone well-versed in keto tell you what to eat, so you don't have to worry about calculating macros or accidentally eating foods that *seem* keto-friendly but turn out not to be.

The only way a diet is going to work long-term is if you like the food you're eating and it leaves you feeling full and satisfied. Trust me, I dieted on and off for years before I found keto.

The number one question I get about keto is "Where do I begin?" The number two question is "What do I eat?!" I love answering these questions because I get to show people how easy keto can be. So for this book, I worked with a nutritionist to put together a one-week meal plan that'll help you with all of that. It's the meal plan I wish I had when I was starting out. It will kickstart ketosis, the food's great, you won't be hungry, and you won't feel overwhelmed trying to plan your own meals. Of course, if you want to plan your own meals, all of the recipes in this book should get you going. But if you just want to jump in, check out the meal plan (page 34).

Try Intermittent Fasting

One way a lot of people make keto work even better is by combining it with intermittent fasting. That's what I do. Without getting too far into it, I'll tell you that it just means eating your meals in a shorter period of time than you normally might. When you do this, it's healthier in a lot of ways because your body isn't spending all day processing food and spiking your insulin levels. Instead, it's using that time to run on the ketone fuel, so you burn fat at a faster rate.

The way I do it is pick a window of like eight hours, and just eat my three meals in that period. So, for instance, I'll eat breakfast at noon, lunch at 3:00, and dinner at 7:30. Boom. You can do it too, and pick whatever window of eight hours you want—like maybe you want to eat breakfast earlier, so then you'll eat dinner earlier, too. Anyway, you can use the meal plan in the next section (or other meals from the book) with or without intermittent fasting. It's up to you, but I wanted to give you options and let you know the way I do it.

My One-Week Meal Plan to Kickstart Ketosis

You can follow this plan to a T or just use it for inspiration. Either way, you'll get yourself going on the right path, and you won't even have to do that much cooking, because we're doing simple meals with lots of leftovers.

	MEAL 1	MEAL 2	MEAL 3	MACROS AND NUTRITION
MONDAY	Traditional Eggs and Bacon Cooked in Butter (page 50)	Loaded Salad Bowl (page 96)	Beef Sausage Meat Loaf (page 194) Coconut Creamed Spinach (page 76)	Fat: 77% Protein: 20% Carbs: 3% Calories: 1256 Total Fat: 108g Total Carbs: 11g Fiber: 4g Net Carbs: 7g Sodium: 765mg Protein: 60g
TUESDAY	Beef Sausage Meat Loaf (leftovers)	Cheesy Garden Veggie Crustless Quiche (page 106)	Simple Flounder in Brown Butter Lemon Sauce (page 126) Tender Grilled Asparagus Spears (page 82)	Fat: 76% Protein: 20% Carbs: 4% Calories: 1228 Total Fat: 104g Total Carbs: 12g Fiber: 3g Net Carbs: 9g Sodium: 836mg Protein: 61g
WEDNESDAY	Hearty Spinach and Bacon Breakfast Bowl (page 57)	Antipasto Salad with Spiralized Zucchini (page 98)	Juicy No-Fail Burger (page 195)	Fat: 75% Protein: 20% Carbs: 5% Calories: 1325 Total Fat: 109g Total Carbs: 23g Fiber: 9g Net Carbs: 14g Sodium: 1285mg Protein: 63g

	MEAL 1	MEAL 2	MEAL 3	MACROS AND NUTRITION
THURSDAY	Super Green Smoothie with Coconut and Raspberries (page 48)	Juicy No-Fail Burger (leftovers) Sautéed Wild Mushrooms with Bacon (page 83)	Chicken Scarpariello with Spicy Sausage (page 146)	Fat: 72% Protein: 22% Carbs: 6% Calories: 1365 Total Fat: 109g Total Carbs: 23g Fiber: 10g Net Carbs: 13g Sodium: 1116mg Protein: 73g
FRIDAY	Creamy Almond Coffee Smoothie (page 46) Hardboiled Eggs with Everything Bagel Seasoning (page 52)	Chicken Scarpariello with Spicy Sausage (leftovers)	New England Clam Chowder (page 88)	Fat: 73% Protein: 20% Carbs: 7% Calories: 1280 Total Fat: 104g Total Carbs: 23g Fiber: 8g Net Carbs: 15g Sodium: 1073mg Protein: 63g
SATURDAY	Italian Sausage Breakfast Casserole (page 60)	New England Clam Chowder (leftovers)	Lemon-Infused Pork Rib Roast (page 176) Simple Butter-Sautéed Vegetables (page 78)	Fat: 72% Protein: 23% Carbs: 5% Calories: 1274 Total Fat: 102g Total Carbs: 16g Fiber: 3g Net Carbs: 13g Sodium: 948mg Protein: 73g
SUNDAY	Golden Pancakes (page 55)	Italian Sausage Breakfast Casserole (leftovers)	Lemon-Infused Pork Rib Roast (leftovers) Simple Butter-Sautéed Vegetables (page 78)	Fat: 74% Protein: 20% Carbs: 6% Calories: 1282 Total Fat: 106g Total Carbs: 22g Fiber: 9g Net Carbs: 13g Sodium: 835mg Protein: 60g

◊Note that this meal plan makes enough for four people because I want you to have leftovers and be able to share the greatness of keto with others.

SNACKS: avocado, beef jerky (sugar-free and low-sodium), berries with whipped coconut cream, celery filled with natural almond butter, handful of pecans, hardboiled eggs, olives

Shopping List

Dairy and Eggs

- Asiago cheese, 2 ounces
- Butter, grass-fed, 1 cup
- Eggs, 27
- Goat cheese, 5 ounces
- Heavy (whipping) cream, 3 cups
- Parmesan cheese, grated, ¾ cup

Meat

- Bacon, uncured, 1¼ pounds (about 20 strips)
- Chicken breasts, boneless, 2 (4-ounce)
- Chicken thighs, boneless, 1 pound
- Flounder fillets, boneless, 4 (4-ounce)
- Genoa salami, 2 ounces
- Ground beef, grass-fed, 2 pounds
- Italian sausage, 3 pounds
- Pepperoni, 1 ounce
- Pork rib roast, 2½ pounds, 4 bones
- Prosciutto, 1 ounce

Produce

- Arugula, 4 cups
- Asparagus, 1 pound
- Avocado, 2
- Basil, fresh, 1 bunch
- Celery, 1 stalk
- Cherry tomatoes, 1 pint
- Garlic, 9 cloves
- Garlic, minced, 5 tablespoons
- Lemon, 2
- Mushrooms, white, 1 cup sliced
- Onion, 2
- Orange, 1
- Parsley, fresh, 1 bunch
- Pimiento, 1
- Raspberries, ½ cup
- Red bell pepper, 4
- Red onion, 1
- Rosemary, 4 sprigs
- Scallion, 1
- Spinach, 1¼ pounds
- Thyme, fresh, 2 bunches
- Tomato, 1
- Wild mushrooms, 4 cups sliced
- Yellow bell pepper, 1
- Zucchini, 4

Pantry items

- Almond butter
- Almond flour
- Arrowroot starch
- Baking powder
- Bay leaves
- Chia seeds
- Cinnamon, ground
- Coconut flour
- Coconut oil
- Coconut water
- Coffee
- Flaxseed meal
- Freshly ground black pepper
- Garlic flakes
- Monk fruit sweetener
- Nutmeg, ground
- Olive oil
- Olive oil cooking spray
- Onion flakes
- Oregano, dried
- Parsley, dried
- Pecans, chopped
- Poppy seeds
- Red pepper flakes
- Sea salt
- Sesame seeds, black
- Sesame seeds, golden
- Vanilla extract

Canned and bottled items

- Almond milk, unsweetened, 3 cups
- Artichokes, marinated, ½ cup
- Chicken stock, 5¼ cups
- Clams, 3 (6½-ounce) cans
- Coconut cream, ¼ cup
- Coconut milk, 2 cups
- Kalamata olives, ¼ cup
- Ranch dressing, ¼ cup
- Vegetable broth, ½ cup
- Worcestershire sauce, 1 teaspoon

Other

- Vanilla protein powder, 2 scoops
- White wine, ¼ cup

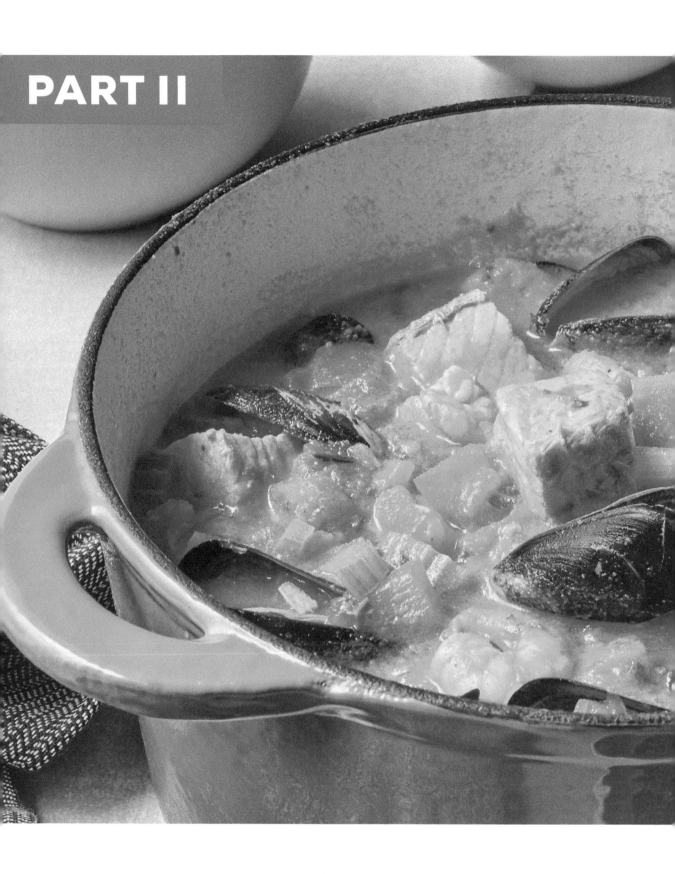

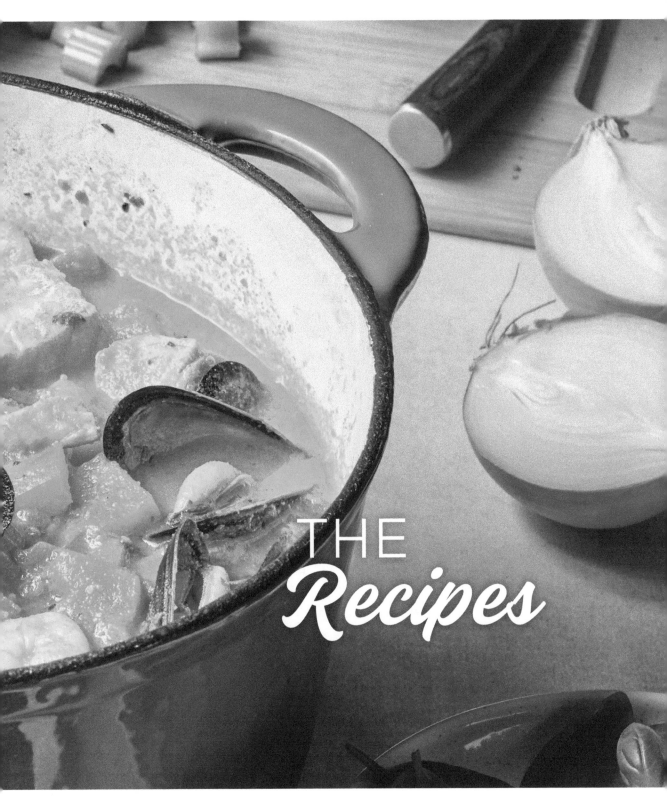

PART II

THE
Recipes

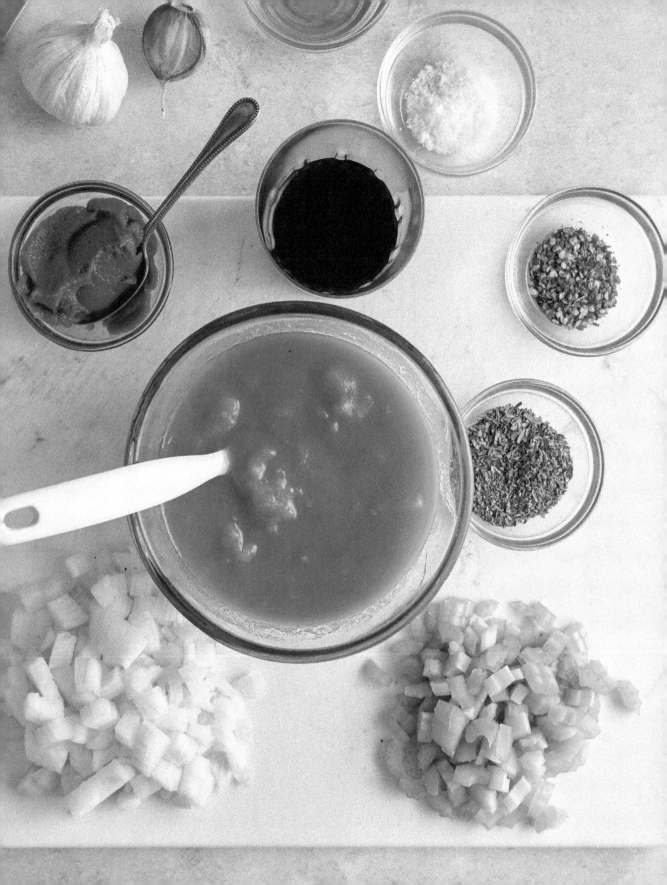

Here are 102 of my absolute favorite keto recipes. What you're going to find here are a lot of easy choices for every meal, whether you just need something to eat by yourself at home or for when you're hosting your entire family. These recipes are clean and healthy, but they have enough fat in them that they're delicious, too (remember: clean, not lean!). My recipes are relatively light on dairy, and obviously there are no grains. In terms of dessert, as I've mentioned a few times, I try to stick to monk fruit when I need a little sweetness. I know these recipes will keep you happy, healthy, and totally satisfied—and make you love eating keto as much as I do.

Special Keto Ingredients

In the recipe chapters, you're going to see some ingredients you might not be familiar with. They might sound weird to you, but you should try them and see how you like them. You might be surprised. Here are some things you'll encounter, with a few notes from me:

- arrowroot (the flour and starch are basically the same, so you can use them interchangeably)
- black sesame seeds (they taste different from regular sesame seeds)
- chia seeds (they have a weird texture, but trust me)
- duck fat (can be used as a delicious replacement for butter if you're avoiding dairy or for other fats/oils you used before you went keto, like margarine)

- flaxseed meal (a good source of fiber and a good replacement for bread crumbs)
- monk fruit sweetener (comes in granulated, powdered, or liquid form, so make sure you note which one the recipe calls for)
- nutritional yeast (can add a cheesy flavor if you prefer less dairy, like me)
- tahini (adds rich flavor and is really healthy)

Note: Sometimes people make comments that keto is expensive. It's true that some of these items aren't cheap, but think about what else you spend your money on. Isn't being healthy and fit important enough to spend some money on? You only get one body. Remember that you are renovating your mind and your kitchen items; if you eliminate all the junk food and takeout, and stick to good-quality food instead, you'll probably end up saving money.

What to Know about Other Ingredients

- As mentioned earlier in the book, all of the meat, eggs, and dairy products you use should be grass-fed, cage-free, hormone-free, and organic. This ensures that you're not ingesting harmful chemicals or weird non-keto additives. Similarly, the bacon you use should be uncured and sugar-free.
- Speaking of dairy, a lot of keto folks like eating dairy because it's tasty and it can be a good way to take in fat. As I've talked about in this book, I don't eat a ton of it, so what I've done here is include some dairy—more than I typically eat—but I've also added tips here and there for making those recipes dairy-free if you want to. Taking out dairy will adjust your macro counts, so just be aware of that.
- You'll see that in these recipes I often call for "good-quality" olive oil. When I say this, I generally mean extra-virgin olive oil or an oil that is meant for eating rather than simply greasing a pan. I leave it to you to decide what olive oil you prefer, though. I also call for "good-quality" in other places, like for cocoa powder and coffee. In places where it makes a difference, I've suggested brands that I like. In other instances, I leave it to you to decide what you like best and what works for your budget.

What to Know about Equipment

- I love grilling, so a lot of these recipes call for a grill. As mentioned in the equipment section, you can use either an outdoor BBQ grill like me, or you can easily use an indoor gas grill or grill pan on your stovetop. It won't make a difference to the recipe instructions.
- I've recently gotten really into using an air fryer. Most of the time, people use air fryers to cut fat from a recipe. That's not why I do it. With keto, you don't want to cut fat from recipes, but I've discovered that an air fryer is a great way to make some foods really crispy and crunchy, which can be hard to achieve on keto because traditional frying isn't really an option (due to the bad oils that are usually used). So you'll see that for some of these recipes I've added a tip about which ones might be great to crisp up with an air fryer. Just be sure to include extra fat in the meal if you do use an air fryer, to keep your macro count right.

What to Know about Recipe Labels

To make things easy, I've included labels on the recipes.

Super Quick: takes 30 minutes or less to make, including prep and cook time

Full Guido: Italian comfort foods and classics remade keto-style

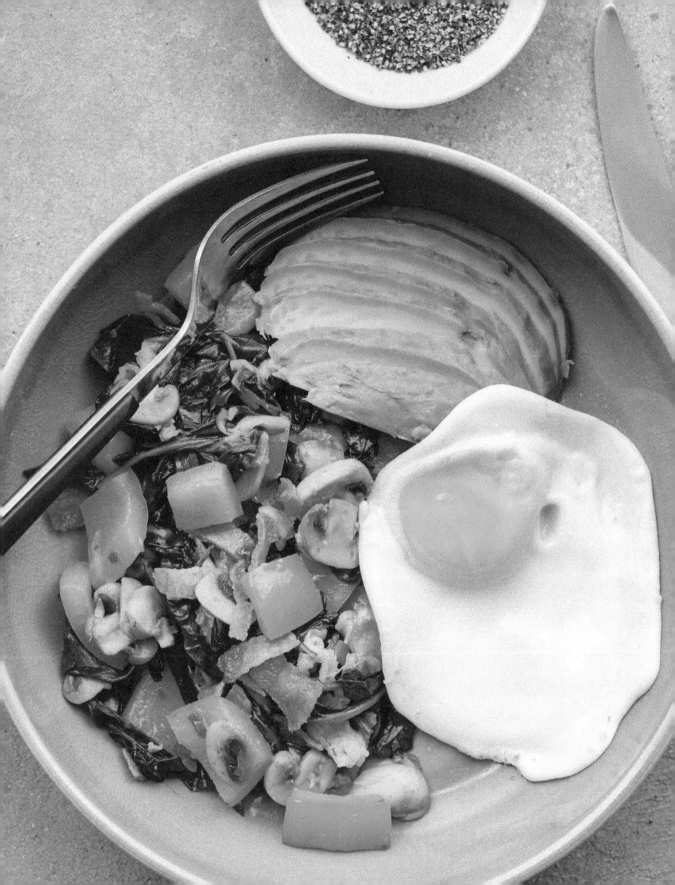

3

Eggs and Breakfast Foods

Breakfast is the first meal I learned to cook. My mom taught me some basics when I was in elementary school, and I've been cooking up eggs ever since. Back then, I used to eat my eggs with a whole pile of toast, so I've had to rethink breakfast so it doesn't include grains. Honestly, the way I was eating—and the way most people eat breakfasts that are filled with carbs—it might as well be dessert! The breakfast foods in this chapter are not like that. They are healthy and will make you feel light as a feather. They'll cut any grogginess because you won't start your day in a carb coma.

Hearty Spinach and Bacon Breakfast Bowl

CREAMY ALMOND COFFEE SMOOTHIE

SUPER QUICK

PREP TIME: 5 MINUTES, PLUS COFFEE FREEZING TIME

SERVES: 2

Keto means giving up your Frappuccinos and other sugary coffee drinks, but with my creamy almond coffee smoothie, you won't miss 'em. This smoothie doesn't just taste good, it also has a lot of great benefits, no matter when you drink it. In the morning, the caffeine will boost your metabolism and get your day off to a great start. If you drink it before a workout, it'll give you a little energy boost to help you power through. Just make sure to use good-quality coffee for the best results.

2 cups strong-brewed coffee

1 cup unsweetened almond milk

1 cup unsweetened coconut milk

2 tablespoons chia seeds

2 tablespoons flax-seed meal

2 tablespoons coconut oil

⅛ teaspoon ground cinnamon

Monk fruit sweetener, granulated, to taste

1. **Make coffee ice cubes.** Pour the coffee into an ice cube tray and freeze for 4 hours minimum.

2. **Blend the smoothie.** Put all of the coffee ice cubes (2 cups worth), almond milk, coconut milk, chia seeds, flaxseed meal, coconut oil, and cinnamon in a blender and blend until smooth and creamy.

3. **Add a sweetener.** Add in as much (or as little) sweetener as you like and blend again.

4. **Serve.** Pour into two tall glasses and serve immediately.

Tip: Make several trays of coffee ice cubes ahead of time and keep them in the freezer so you can make this smoothie quickly in the morning. Pop them out of the trays after they have frozen and store them in sealed freezer bags. Two cups of brewed coffee will make about 1 tray of ice cubes.

PER SERVING
Macronutrients: Fat: 88%; Protein: 6%; Carbs: 6%
Calories: 444; Total fat: 44g; Total carbs: 6g; Fiber: 4g;
Net carbs: 2g; Sodium: 106mg; Protein: 6g

MOCHA PRE-WORKOUT SMOOTHIE

SUPER QUICK

PREP TIME: 5 MINUTES

SERVES: 2

This is my go-to pre-workout smoothie. When you drink coffee before you exercise, it can get your body burning fat cells as energy instead of glycogen even faster. This recipe smoothie has more carbs than a lot of keto recipes because of the banana, but to me those carbs are worth it for a few reasons. One, bananas help stimulate dopamine production in your brain, which makes you feel good and helps you recover quicker after you exercise. And two, the banana adds some sweetness, which honestly makes this smoothie taste fantastic. Bananas can be controversial in the keto world since they're pretty sweet, but this recipe doesn't call for a lot, and personally I think it's more excusable because you are about to work out. If you'd rather leave the banana out, that's cool, you do you. In my opinion, though, if you're working out hard you earned that little half a banana. You can eat it when your body is in burning mode.

1 cup full-fat coconut milk

1 cup almond milk

2 scoops (25–28 grams) chocolate protein powder (use something with no or very few carbs—I use Primal Fuel)

½ banana

½ cup brewed espresso

1 tablespoon cocoa powder

4 ice cubes

1. **Blend the smoothie.** Put the coconut milk, almond milk, protein powder, banana, espresso, cocoa powder, and ice in a blender and blend until smooth and creamy.

2. **Serve.** Pour into two tall glasses and serve.

Swap: You can use 2 cups of coconut milk instead of almond milk for a super-rich smoothie, especially if you are following strict keto macros. This swap will change the calories to 576 and the macros to Fat: 70%; Protein: 20%; Carbs: 10%.

PER SERVING
Macronutrients: Fat: 63%; Protein: 24%; Carbs: 13%
Calories: 372; Total fat: 27g; Total carbs: 14g; Fiber: 5g;
Net carbs: 9g; Sodium: 381mg; Protein: 26g

SUPER GREEN SMOOTHIE WITH COCONUT AND RASPBERRIES

SUPER QUICK
PREP TIME: 10 MINUTES
SERVES: 2

I love starting my day with this green smoothie because it just makes me *feel* healthy—because it actually is. I'll also drink one when my energy is lagging a little bit and I need a snack to fill me up. There are lots of super healthy green vegetables you can use for this drink, like spinach, kale, chard, beet greens, dandelion, cilantro, and parsley. It's a great reminder that micronutrients are just as important as macronutrients.

2 cups spinach

2 cups unsweetened almond milk

1 cup coconut water

2 scoops (25–28 grams) vanilla protein powder

½ cup fresh parsley

½ cup raspberries

2 tablespoons almond butter

2 tablespoons coconut oil

6 ice cubes

1. **Blend the smoothie.** Put the spinach, almond milk, coconut water, protein powder, parsley, raspberries, almond butter, coconut oil, and ice in a blender and blend until smooth and creamy.

2. **Serve.** Pour into two tall glasses and serve.

Swap: Kale or Swiss chard works very well in this smoothie but they will create an earthier flavor. Use other greens in same amount for best results.

PER SERVING
Macronutrients: Fat: 60%; Protein: 25%; Carbs: 15%
Calories: 401; Total fat: 27g; Total carbs: 16g; Fiber: 8g;
Net carbs: 8g; Sodium: 410mg; Protein: 28g

TAHINI BANANA DETOX SMOOTHIE

SUPER QUICK
PREP TIME: 10 MINUTES
SERVES: 2

If you've never had tahini, you're going to be surprised when you taste this smoothie—in a good way. It's got a super-rich taste, almost a little smoky, and I can't get enough of the stuff. Plus it's a good source of calcium, iron, magnesium, and vitamin B_1. Tahini isn't really sweet, though, which is why I use banana here to balance out the flavor. You may notice that the net carbs for this recipe are higher than I usually go, so this is another smoothie I like to drink before working out when I know I'm about to burn a lot of fuel.

1½ cups unsweetened almond milk

½ cup heavy (whipping) cream

1 banana

2 scoops (25–28 grams) vanilla protein powder

2 tablespoons tahini

½ teaspoon ground cinnamon

5 ice cubes

1. **Blend the smoothie.** Put the almond milk, cream, banana, protein powder, tahini, cinnamon, and ice in a blender and blend until smooth and creamy.

2. **Serve.** Pour into two tall glasses and serve.

Tip: You can increase the tahini by 2 tablespoons if you love the taste. This will add about 90 calories, 8 grams of fat, 3 grams of protein, and 2 net carbs.

PER SERVING
Macronutrients: Fat: 65%; Protein: 20%; Carbs: 15%
Calories: 425; Total fat: 29g; Total carbs: 16g; Fiber: 6g;
Net carbs: 10g; Sodium: 498mg; Protein: 25g

TRADITIONAL EGGS AND BACON COOKED IN BUTTER

SUPER QUICK

PREP TIME: 5 MINUTES | COOK TIME: 15 MINUTES

SERVES: 1

Eggs and bacon is a classic breakfast dish, but this doesn't *have* to be a breakfast food. A perfect fried egg adds so much to a burger or even a salad, so definitely think about this recipe for lunch and dinner, too. In this recipe, I say to use "uncured bacon." That's because it doesn't have the harmful nitrates (and cane sugar) in it like cured bacon. One warning about the bacon, though: It's tempting to just mow down an entire package, but try to pace yourself and eat it in moderate amounts. It has a great fat-to-protein ratio, but it's really high in sodium. Plus, once you have a few slices you will be satiated and won't need a ton more.

1 tablespoon grass-fed butter, divided

2 strips uncured bacon

2 eggs

Sea salt, for seasoning

Freshly ground black pepper, for seasoning

1. **Cook the bacon.** In a large skillet over medium-high heat, melt ½ tablespoon of butter. Add the bacon to the pan and fry until it is cooked through and crispy, turning once, about 10 minutes total. Transfer the bacon to paper towels to drain and wipe the skillet with more paper towels.

2. **Cook the eggs.** Turn the heat down to medium. Add the remaining ½ tablespoon of butter to the skillet. Carefully crack the eggs into the skillet and cook until the whites are completely set, about 3 minutes.

3. **Serve.** Carefully transfer the eggs and bacon to a plate and season the eggs with salt and pepper.

Tip: Don't try to speed up the cooking time on fried eggs with higher temperatures. High heat will change the protein structure of the eggs, making them rubbery with hard brown edges.

PER SERVING
Macronutrients: Fat: 83%; Protein: 16%; Carbs: 1%
Calories: 500; Total fat: 47g; Total carbs: 1g; Fiber: 0g;
Net carbs: 1g; Sodium: 253mg; Protein: 19g

HARDBOILED EGGS WITH EVERYTHING BAGEL SEASONING

SUPER QUICK

PREP TIME: 5 MINUTES | COOK TIME: 15 MINUTES, PLUS COOLING TIME

SERVES: 2

Everything bagel seasoning is one of my best ways to avoid getting bored with the food on keto—it instantly changes and improves the flavor of things like eggs, fish, chicken, and kale chips. (And don't worry, it won't make you crave an actual bagel, though it's also a great little trick to fill the craving, if you do.) When you're making the seasoning for this recipe, add more or less of any of the ingredients depending on your personal taste. Just go with coarser-texture spices because things with finer textures, like onion powder or garlic powder, will get lost in there.

FOR THE SEASONING

3 tablespoons sesame seeds

1 tablespoon black sesame seeds

1 tablespoon onion flakes

2 teaspoons poppy seeds

1 teaspoon garlic flakes

1 teaspoon coarse sea salt

FOR THE EGGS

4 eggs

TO MAKE THE SEASONING

Mix the seasonings. In a small jar with a lid, stir together the sesame seeds, black sesame seeds, onion flakes, poppy seeds, garlic flakes, and salt until everything is well combined. Store in the sealed jar for up to six months.

TO MAKE THE EGGS

1. **Boil the eggs.** In a medium saucepan, carefully place the eggs in a single layer. Add enough water to cover the eggs by about 1 inch. Cover the pan and bring the water to a boil over medium-high heat. Boil for 1 minute, then remove the pan from the heat and let it stand, covered, for 10 minutes.

2. **Cool and peel the eggs.** Remove the eggs from the water with a slotted spoon and run them under cold water to cool them. To peel, tap each egg a few times on a hard surface and carefully pull the shells off the eggs. Give the eggs a quick rinse under cool water to remove any remaining bits of shell.

3. **Season and serve.** Sprinkle the eggs with some seasoning and divide the eggs between two plates.

Tip: Hardboiled eggs make a great snack, so double the recipe in a larger saucepan and store the cooled eggs for up to one week in the refrigerator. Just make sure you mark the hardboiled eggs on their shell with a pen so you know which are raw and which are cooked.

PER SERVING
Macronutrients: Fat: 65%; Protein: 26%; Carbs: 9%
Calories: 235; Total fat: 17g; Total carbs: 6g; Fiber: 2g;
Net carbs: 4g; Sodium: 422mg; Protein: 15g

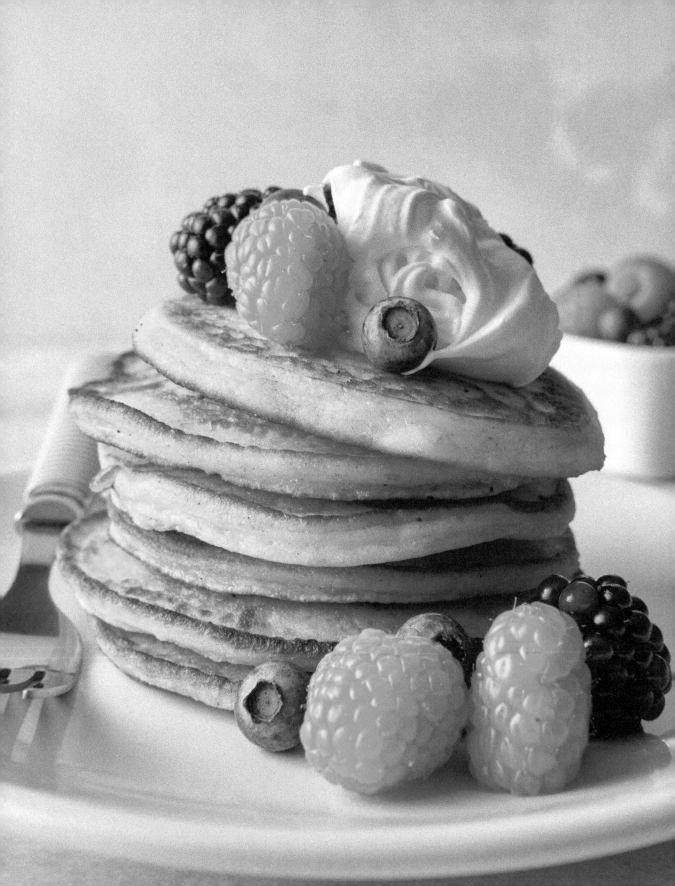

GOLDEN PANCAKES

SUPER QUICK

PREP TIME: 5 MINUTES | COOK TIME: 20 MINUTES

SERVES: 4

I was so happy when I perfected this recipe because I missed pancakes once I started doing keto—and I like these even more than the unhealthy pancakes I used to eat. I don't just eat these at breakfast, either. I've had them for every meal and even eaten them cold as a snack by throwing a little almond butter on top. The key is to get the batter to a traditional "pancake batter" consistency when you add the liquid. And if you use syrup or another sweet ingredient like berries as a topping, don't use the monk fruit sweetener. If you're gonna follow the Keto Guido way of doing things, I give you permission to find a low sugar/carb natural syrup—just don't make it an everyday thing. Remember, this is a lifestyle, not a prison sentence.

⅔ cup almond flour

⅓ cup coconut flour

1 tablespoon monk fruit sweetener, powder form (optional)

1 teaspoon baking powder

¼ teaspoon ground nutmeg

3 eggs

¼ to ½ cup coconut milk

3 tablespoons coconut oil

1 teaspoon pure vanilla extract

Grass-fed butter, for cooking the pancakes

½ cup sugar-free syrup (optional)

1. **Mix the dry ingredients.** In a large bowl, stir together the almond flour, coconut flour, monk fruit sweetener (if using), baking powder, and nutmeg until everything is well blended.

2. **Add the wet ingredients.** In a small bowl, whisk together the eggs, ¼ cup of the coconut milk, and the coconut oil and vanilla. Add the wet ingredients to the dry ingredients and whisk until the batter is smooth. If the batter is too thick, add more coconut milk.

CONTINUED ▶

3. **Cook the pancakes.** In a large skillet over medium heat, melt the butter. Drop the pancake batter by tablespoons, about 3 per pancake, and spread it out to form circles. You should be able to cook about four pancakes per batch. Cook until bubbles form on the pancakes and burst, about 2 minutes. Flip the pancakes and cook until browned and cooked through, about 2 more minutes. Transfer the pancakes to a plate and set it aside. Repeat with the remaining batter until it's all used up.

4. **Serve.** Divide the pancakes between four plates and top with your favorite accompaniments.

Tip: These golden beauties are delicious with sugar-free syrup, fresh berries, nut butter, whipped cream, cream cheese, toasted nuts, or butter.

Ditch the Dairy: Cook the pancakes with 1 tablespoon of coconut oil instead of the butter.

PER SERVING (3 PANCAKES)
Macronutrients: Fat: 75%; Protein: 13%; Carbs: 12%
Calories: 389; Total fat: 33g; Total carbs: 14g; Fiber: 8g;
Net carbs: 4g; Sodium: 118mg; Protein: 10g

HEARTY SPINACH AND BACON BREAKFAST BOWL

SUPER QUICK

PREP TIME: 10 MINUTES | COOK TIME: 10 MINUTES

SERVES: 2

Breakfast bowls are my go-to on days when I need something filling and nutritious but don't have much time. This is great for using your leftovers because you can sub in stuff you've got in your fridge, like chicken, Cheddar, ground beef, or cauliflower. If you want to get even more energy from this, add a fried or poached egg on top.

1 tablespoon coconut oil

2 red bell peppers, chopped

½ cup sliced white mushrooms

1 teaspoon minced garlic

½ teaspoon red pepper flakes

4 cups chopped spinach, thoroughly washed

8 cooked uncured bacon slices, chopped

½ cup grated Asiago cheese

½ avocado, sliced

1. **Sauté the vegetables.** In a large skillet over medium-high heat, melt the coconut oil. Add the red bell peppers, mushrooms, garlic, and red pepper flakes and sauté them until they've softened, about 3 minutes. Add the spinach and cook until it has wilted, about 4 minutes.

2. **Finish cooking.** Stir in the bacon and Asiago and cook for 2 minutes more.

3. **Serve.** Divide the mixture between four bowls and top with the avocado slices.

Tip: Save the bacon fat after cooking to use in other recipes. It's a great alternative to butter or coconut oil and adds a richness to almost any finished dish.

Ditch the Dairy: Leave out the Asiago, and instead increase the bacon to 10 slices and cook them first in the skillet. Remove the cooked bacon and cook the vegetables in the bacon fat in the skillet. This will increase the fat and protein in this dish.

PER SERVING
Macronutrients: Fat: 65%; Protein: 25%; Carbs: 10%
Calories: 445; Total fat: 32g; Total carbs: 14g; Fiber: 6g;
Net carbs: 8g; Sodium: 224mg; Protein: 26g

VEGETABLE-BEEF HASH WITH NESTED EGGS

FULL GUIDO

PREP TIME: 5 MINUTES | COOK TIME: 35 MINUTES

SERVES: 4

Once you try these eggs, it may be hard for you to go back to eating eggs any other way. Eggs cook beautifully in sauces, and these will turn out flavorful and tender. I use grass-fed beef because it has twice as many omega-3 fatty acids as grain-fed beef. In this recipe I use 85 percent lean beef, but if you want to use beef with more fat in it, that works, too.

2 tablespoons good-quality olive oil

½ pound grass-fed ground beef

½ red bell pepper, diced

½ zucchini, diced

¼ onion, diced

2 teaspoons minced garlic

1½ cups low-carb tomato sauce

1 tablespoon dried basil

1 teaspoon dried oregano

⅛ teaspoon sea salt

⅛ teaspoon freshly ground black pepper

4 eggs

1. **Cook the beef.** In a large deep skillet over medium-high heat, warm the olive oil. Add the beef and, stirring it occasionally, cook until it is completely browned, about 10 minutes.

2. **Make the sauce.** Add the bell pepper, zucchini, onion, and garlic to the skillet and sauté for 3 minutes. Stir in the tomato sauce, basil, oregano, salt, and pepper, bring it to a boil, and cook for about 10 minutes.

3. **Cook the eggs.** Make four wells in the beef mixture using the back of a spoon. Crack an egg into each well, then cover the skillet, reduce the heat to medium-low, and simmer until the eggs are cooked through, about 10 minutes.

4. **Serve.** Divide the mixture between four bowls, making sure to include an egg in each serving.

Swap: The ground beef can be replaced with the same amount of hot or mild Italian sausage or even ground chicken for a different flavor. The chicken will not contain as much fat so you can add a sprinkle of cheese (whatever kind you like) on top.

PER SERVING
Macronutrients: Fat: 65%; Protein: 25%; Carbs: 10%
Calories: 275; Total fat: 19g; Total carbs: 8g; Fiber: 2g;
Net carbs: 6g; Sodium: 141mg; Protein: 18g

ITALIAN SAUSAGE BREAKFAST CASSEROLE

FULL GUIDO

PREP TIME: 5 MINUTES | COOK TIME: 40 MINUTES

SERVES: 6

I call this a casserole, but it's really kind of like a frittata—you're just cooking it casserole-style here. My typical Sicilian family usually needs a loaf of bread with their food, but I made this for them once and they licked their plates clean . . . and didn't even know they were eating keto!

Olive oil cooking spray

1 pound hot or mild Italian sausage

6 eggs

¾ cup grated Parmesan cheese

½ red bell pepper, chopped

½ cup coconut milk

¼ cup Spinach Basil Pesto (page 224)

1 tablespoon chopped fresh basil

1. **Preheat the oven.** Set the oven temperature to 400°F. Lightly grease an 8-by-8-inch baking dish with olive oil cooking spray.

2. **Cook the sausage.** In a large skillet over medium-high heat, cook the sausage, breaking it up with a spoon while it cooks, until it's lightly browned, about 10 minutes. Spread the sausage evenly over the bottom of the baking dish.

3. **Mix the remaining ingredients.** In a medium bowl, whisk together the eggs, Parmesan, red bell pepper, coconut milk, and pesto. Pour the mixture over the sausage.

4. **Bake the casserole.** Bake for 30 minutes or until it's cooked through and lightly golden and puffy.

5. **Serve.** Sprinkle the basil over the casserole and serve.

Tip: The casserole can be completely put together through step 3, covered with plastic wrap, and stored in the refrigerator for up to 12 hours. Pop it in the oven and bake for 45 minutes at 400°F. This can save time and cleanup if you make it the night before a breakfast gathering.

Ditch the Dairy: Leave out the Parmesan, and instead increase the sausage to 1¼ pounds to increase the fat and protein in this dish.

PER SERVING
Macronutrients: Fat: 76%; Protein: 20%; Carbs: 4%
Calories: 408; Total fat: 34g; Total carbs: 3g; Fiber: 0g;
Net carbs: 3g; Sodium: 537mg; Protein: 19g

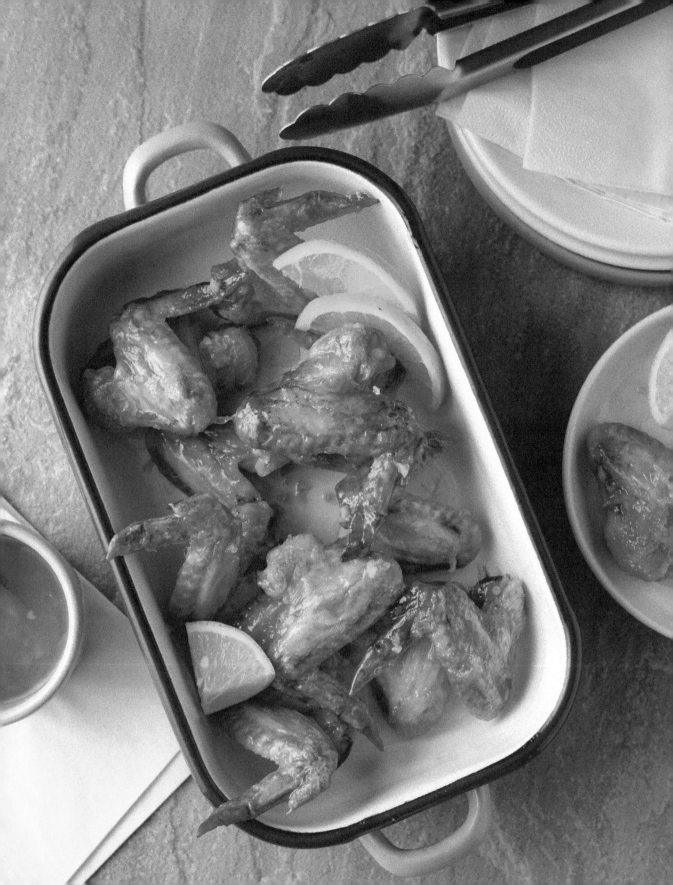

Snacks and Sides

One of the most frequent questions I get about keto is "What snacks can I eat?" Those of us that are American were all raised in a snack-oriented world. Snacks are almost more important to people these days than real food, and you can tell because everywhere you look, you see all this processed junk on the shelves. I think because our snacks are so high in carbohydrates, they keep us hungry so we always need to eat more snacks (chips, soda, candy, etc.). But as you know from the first part of the book, my philosophy is that eating real whole foods keeps you satiated so you don't need to eat so many snacks. That being said, I know that you might need a pick-me-up from time to time between meals, so these are my snacks that are made of real food and serve a nutritional purpose.

HOT CHARD ARTICHOKE DIP

SUPER QUICK

PREP TIME: 10 MINUTES | COOK TIME: 20 MINUTES
SERVES: 4

If you're looking for a dip for when people are coming over, or if you just want one for a snack, this dip is quick, easy, and amazing. You can also mix it all up and refrigerate it a few days before, and then bake it right before the party.

4 ounces cream cheese, at room temperature

½ cup coconut milk

½ cup grated Asiago cheese

½ cup shredded Cheddar cheese

1 teaspoon minced garlic

Dash hot sauce (optional)

2 cups chopped Swiss chard

½ cup roughly chopped artichoke hearts (packed in brine, not oil)

1. **Preheat the oven.** Set the oven temperature to 450°F.

2. **Mix the ingredients.** In a large bowl, stir together the cream cheese, coconut milk, Asiago, Cheddar, garlic, and hot sauce (if using), until everything is well mixed. Stir in the chard and the artichoke hearts and mix until they're well incorporated. **Note:** You've got to use artichokes packed in brine rather than oil because the extra oil will come out of the dip when you heat it, which will mess up the texture.

3. **Bake.** Spoon the mixture into a 1-quart baking dish, and bake it for 15 to 20 minutes until it's bubbly and lightly golden.

4. **Serve.** Cut up low-carb veggies to serve with this creamy, rich dip.

Tip: Some low-carb vegetables that are great with this dip include broccoli, asparagus, mushrooms, zucchini, and radishes.

Swap: Kale or spinach will also be delicious instead of Swiss chard. If using kale, you'll want to blanch the leaves first to make them less tough. To blanch: Remove the stems, then dunk the leaves in boiling water. Leave them there for about 3 minutes, then remove them and run them under cold water or put them in a bowl filled with ice water.

PER SERVING
Macronutrients: Fat: 77%; Protein: 17%; Carbs: 6%
Calories: 280; Total fat: 25g; Total carbs: 5g; Fiber: 1g;
Net carbs: 4g; Sodium: 411mg; Protein: 11g

CHEESE ALMOND CRACKERS

SUPER QUICK

PREP TIME: 10 MINUTES | COOK TIME: 20 MINUTES

SERVES: 4

As much as I love keto, when I was starting out, I did miss "the crunch." You know what I mean—the one you get from the chips, pretzels, and crackers. Luckily, I discovered I could still get it by making these Cheese Almond Crackers. These are perfect for when you just want a crispy cracker with cheese or to use with a dip. The nutritional yeast in there sounds weird, but it adds a cheesy flavor that I like. And honestly, you can do anything with crackers. Being Italian, one of my favorite dishes is cold antipasto (prosciutto, cheese, and olives), but to make it complete, you need some sort of bread, which is where this comes in handy. A little cracker on the side will fill that craving if you feel the need for "the crunch" or a piece of bread.

Olive oil cooking spray

1 cup almond flour

½ cup finely shredded Cheddar cheese

1 tablespoon nutritional yeast

¼ teaspoon baking soda

¼ teaspoon garlic powder

¼ teaspoon sea salt

1 egg

2 teaspoons good-quality olive oil

1. **Preheat the oven.** Set the oven temperature to 350°F. Line a baking sheet with parchment paper and set it aside. Lightly grease two sheets of parchment paper with olive oil cooking spray and set them aside.

2. **Mix the dry ingredients.** In a large bowl, stir together the almond flour, Cheddar, nutritional yeast, baking soda, garlic powder, and salt until everything is well blended.

3. **Mix the wet ingredients.** In a small bowl, whisk together the egg and olive oil. Using a wooden spoon, mix the wet ingredients into the dry until the dough sticks together to form a ball. Gather the ball together using your hands, and knead it firmly a few times.

4. **Roll out the dough.** Place the ball on one of the lightly greased parchment paper pieces and press it down to form a disk. Place the other piece of greased parchment paper on top and use a rolling pin to roll the dough into a 9-by-12-inch rectangle about ⅛ inch thick.

5. **Cut the dough.** Use a pizza cutter and a ruler to cut the edges of the dough into an even rectangle and cut the dough into 1½-by-1½-inch columns and rows. Transfer the crackers to the baking sheet.

6. **Bake.** Bake the crackers for 15 to 20 minutes until they're crisp. Transfer them to a wire rack and let them cool completely.

7. **Serve.** Eat the crackers immediately or store them in an airtight container in the refrigerator for up to one week.

Swap: The seasonings for these crackers can be varied so be bold and try flaxseeds, sesame, rosemary, thyme, and anything else you enjoy.

Alternative method: Use an air fryer to crisp these up. Instead of baking, air fry the crackers at 400°F. Spray the air fryer basket with the olive oil cooking spray (do not use baking spray as it may damage the air fryer basket, but also because you don't want to ingest that bad stuff). Place the crackers in the basket in a single layer. Air fry for 8 minutes, and then shake the basket gently and cook for another 4 to 5 minutes until the crackers are light golden brown. Cool on a wire rack. Repeat with the remaining dough.

PER SERVING
Macronutrients: Fat: 75%; Protein: 21%; Carbs: 4%
Calories: 146; Total fat: 12g; Total carbs: 1g; Fiber: 1g;
Net carbs: 0g; Sodium: 105mg; Protein: 7g

CRAB STUFFED MUSHROOMS

SUPER QUICK

PREP TIME: 10 MINUTES | COOK TIME: 20 MINUTES

SERVES: 4

Crab stuffed mushrooms are a classic appetizer in the non-keto world that translate over beautifully to keto. The flavors here just work so well together. When you're making this recipe, remember to drain the mushrooms well so you don't get hit with hot juices shooting out when you bite into them. This recipe is a good one to try at your next party or special dinner.

1 cup cooked chopped crab

1 cup cream cheese, softened

½ cup grated Parmesan cheese

¼ cup ground almonds

1 scallion, chopped

1 tablespoon chopped fresh parsley

1 teaspoon minced garlic

12 large button mushrooms, cleaned and stemmed

Olive oil cooking spray

1. **Preheat the oven.** Set the oven temperature to 375°F. Line a baking sheet with parchment paper.

2. **Mix the filling.** In a large bowl, stir together the crab, cream cheese, Parmesan, almonds, scallion, parsley, and garlic until everything is well mixed.

3. **Precook the mushrooms.** Place the mushrooms stem-side up on the baking sheet and lightly spray them with olive oil. Bake them for 2 minutes then drain them stem-side down on paper towels.

4. **Stuff the mushrooms.** Turn the mushrooms over and place them back on the baking sheet. Spoon about 1½ tablespoons of the filling into each mushroom.

5. **Bake the mushrooms.** Bake for 15 minutes until the mushrooms are lightly golden and bubbly.

6. **Serve.** Arrange the mushrooms on a serving platter.

Tip: You can prepare the mushrooms through step 4 and store them in the refrigerator for up to two days in a sealed container until you want to bake them.

PER SERVING
Macronutrients: Fat: 72%; Protein: 22%; Carbs: 6%
Calories: 300; Total fat: 25g; Total carbs: 4g; Fiber: 0g;
Net carbs: 4g; Sodium: 554mg; Protein: 16g

SMOKED SALMON CREAM CHEESE ROLLUPS WITH ARUGULA AND TRUFFLE OIL DRIZZLE

SUPER QUICK
PREP TIME: 10 MINUTES
SERVES: 4

Smoked salmon is a really good choice for keto because it's high in protein, low in carbs, and filled with omega-3 fatty acids, B vitamins, vitamin A, and vitamin D. And when you eat it with cream cheese, arugula, and truffle oil, it's one of those moments when you won't believe this counts as a "diet." I also just love truffle oil—it makes this quick snack taste like you're eating at a five-star restaurant.

½ cup cream cheese

¼ cup plain Greek-style yogurt

2 teaspoons chopped fresh dill

12 slices (½ pound) smoked salmon

¾ cup arugula

Truffle oil, for garnish

1. **Mix the filling.** In a small bowl, blend together the cream cheese, yogurt, and dill until the mixture is smooth.

2. **Make the rollups.** Spread the cream cheese mixture onto the smoked salmon slices, dividing it evenly. Place several arugula leaves at one end of each slice and roll them up. Secure them with a toothpick if they're starting to unroll.

3. **Serve.** Drizzle the rolls with truffle oil and place three rolls on each of four plates.

Tip: Be very sparing when drizzling the truffle oil because it can overpower all the other flavors in the dish. Look for truffle-infused olive oil rather than synthetic oils for the best taste and quality.

PER SERVING
Macronutrients: Fat: 74%; Protein: 23%; Carbs: 3%
Calories: 234; Total fat: 20g; Total carbs: 2g; Fiber: 0g;
Net carbs: 2g; Sodium: 540mg; Protein: 13g

WARM HERBED OLIVES

SUPER QUICK | FULL GUIDO

PREP TIME: 5 MINUTES | COOK TIME: 4 MINUTES

SERVES: 4

I love olives. Obviously, being from an Italian family, I grew up eating them all the time, and I'm happy that I can still enjoy them on keto. The good news is they're also really healthy. They've been connected to a lower risk of heart disease and they're great for your skin. In this recipe, I use thyme, fennel seeds, and red pepper flakes for seasoning, but really, you can use any herbs or spices depending on what you like.

¼ cup good-quality olive oil

4 ounces green olives

4 ounces Kalamata olives

½ teaspoon dried thyme

¼ teaspoon fennel seeds

Pinch red pepper flakes

1. **Sauté the olives.** In a large skillet over medium heat, warm the olive oil. Sauté the olives, thyme, fennel seeds, and red pepper flakes until the olives start to brown, 3 to 4 minutes.

2. **Serve.** Put the olives into a bowl and serve them warm.

Tip: You can use pitted olives for this snack if you want to avoid having to pit them while eating.

Swap: Any type of olive will work in this dish. You can also add sundried tomatoes and artichoke hearts for a tasty variation. One tablespoon of these variations per serving will add about 1 gram of carbs.

PER SERVING (¼ CUP)
Macronutrients: Fat: 92%; Protein: 1%; Carbs: 7%
Calories: 165; Total fat: 17g; Total carbs: 3g; Fiber: 1g;
Net carbs: 2g; Sodium: 503mg; Protein: 1g

CHICKEN WINGS WITH ORANGE-GINGER SAUCE

PREP TIME: 5 MINUTES | COOK TIME: 40 MINUTES
SERVES: 4

Chicken wings are like the ultimate comfort food. They're crispy, they're satisfying, and they're delicious no matter what you're doing—hanging out with friends on the patio, watching sports, eating them cold for lunch the next day, whatever. My wings use a special orange-ginger sauce you're going to love. It has a nice flair to it with just a little bite, and you're going to want to sprinkle a few sesame seeds on them to get the full effect. If you want your wings extra crispy, check out the air fryer tip below.

FOR THE WINGS
2 pounds chicken wings

2 tablespoons coconut oil, melted

FOR THE SAUCE
4 tablespoons grass-fed butter

2 teaspoons grated fresh ginger

2 teaspoons minced garlic

Zest and juice of 1 orange

2 tablespoons monk fruit sweetener, granulated form

TO MAKE THE WINGS

1. **Preheat the oven.** Set the oven temperature to 400°F. Line a baking sheet with parchment paper.

2. **Prepare the wings.** In a large bowl, toss the wings with the coconut oil and spread them on the baking sheet.

3. **Bake the wings.** Bake the wings for 20 minutes, turn them over, and bake them for another 20 minutes until they're golden and cooked through (165°F internal temperature).

TO MAKE THE SAUCE

1. **Make the sauce.** While the chicken wings are baking, put a small saucepan over medium-high heat and melt the butter. Add the ginger and garlic and sauté for 3 minutes. Stir in the orange zest, orange juice, and monk fruit sweetener and bring the sauce to a boil. Reduce the heat to medium and simmer, stirring from time to time, until the sauce gets thick and shiny, 10 to 15 minutes.

2. **Glaze the wings.** Transfer the wings to a large bowl and pour in the sauce, tossing the wings to coat them completely. Serve with lots of napkins.

Swap: You can make the basic wing recipe here and replace the sauce with whatever suits your taste, like butter and garlic, keto barbeque sauce, or even simply toss them with salt and pepper.

Alternative method: This is a great recipe to use an air fryer with to crisp these up even more. In that case, instead of baking the wings, air fry them at 350°F. Spray the basket with olive oil cooking spray. Remove the chicken wings from the marinade. Toss in ½ cup of almond flour. Preheat the air fryer for 3 minutes. Add half of the wings to the air fryer and cook for 15 minutes. Shake the basket and cook for another 13 minutes. Increase the air fryer temperature to 400°F and cook for 6 to 7 minutes longer until the wings reach 165°F internally. Repeat with the remaining wings. If you want to serve them all at once, add the first batch back to the air fryer with the second batch and cook for 1 to 2 minutes at 400°F until hot.

PER SERVING
Macronutrients: Fat: 72%; Protein: 26%; Carbs: 2%
Calories: 674; Total fat: 54g; Total carbs: 3g; Fiber: 0g;
Net carbs: 3g; Sodium: 274mg; Protein: 42g

CRISPY GRILLED KALE LEAVES

SUPER QUICK

PREP TIME: 10 MINUTES | COOK TIME: 5 MINUTES

SERVES: 4

I'll be real with you: I don't always love kale straight up. But when I grill it, it gets this great smoky flavor and a crunchy texture that makes me crave it. And I'm glad I found a way to make it so delicious because kale is kind of a miracle vegetable. It's one of the healthiest foods in the world because it's loaded with antioxidants, so it's perfect for a guilt-free snack.

½ cup good-quality olive oil

2 teaspoons freshly squeezed lemon juice

½ teaspoon garlic powder

7 cups large kale leaves, thoroughly washed and patted dry

Sea salt, for seasoning

Freshly ground black pepper, for seasoning

1. **Preheat the grill.** Set the grill to medium-high heat.

2. **Mix the dressing.** In a large bowl, whisk together the olive oil, lemon juice, and garlic powder until it thickens.

3. **Prepare the kale.** Add the kale leaves to the bowl and use your fingers to massage the dressing thoroughly all over the leaves. Season the leaves lightly with salt and pepper.

4. **Grill and serve.** Place the kale leaves in a single layer on the preheated grill. Grill for 1 to 2 minutes, turn the leaves over, and grill the other side for 1 minute, until they're crispy. Put the leaves on a platter and serve.

Swap: Instead of garlic powder you can season the crispy kale with your favorite herbs and spices. Add the seasonings after grilling because some additions can develop an unpleasant flavor when heated too much. Try paprika, cumin, coriander, or chili.

Alternative method: This is a great recipe to use an air fryer with to crisp these up even more. In that case, instead of baking the kale, air fry it at 370°F. Tear the kale leaves into 2 or 3 pieces each. Add the dressing and seasonings. Spray the basket with olive oil cooking spray. Drain the excess marinade from the kale. Add half of the kale to the basket and cook for 6 minutes. Shake the basket and cook for 2 to 4 minutes longer until they're slightly crisp; they will crisp up more as they cool. Cool them in a single layer on a wire rack. Repeat with the remaining kale.

PER SERVING
Macronutrients: Fat: 86%; Protein: 3%; Carbs: 11%
Calories: 282; Total fat: 28g; Total carbs: 9g; Fiber: 3g;
Net carbs: 6g; Sodium: 37mg; Protein: 3g

COCONUT CREAMED SPINACH

SUPER QUICK

PREP TIME: 10 MINUTES | COOK TIME: 20 MINUTES

SERVES: 4

Creamed vegetables are a true comfort food because, if you're like me, they instantly take you back to the big, loud family meals from when you were a kid, everyone sitting around, with huge bowls and platters on the table, and creamed vegetables were always in there. My coconut creamed spinach is a more evolved version of what we used to eat back then, but it still tastes so good. I love eating at steakhouses, and my favorite side dish there is always the creamed spinach. So when I crave it at home, this is my go-to.

1 tablespoon
  grass-fed butter

¼ onion, thinly sliced

4 cups coarsely
  chopped spinach,
  thoroughly washed

½ cup vegetable broth

¼ cup coconut cream

⅛ teaspoon
  ground nutmeg

Pinch sea salt

Pinch freshly ground
  black pepper

1. **Cook the onion.** In a large skillet over medium heat, melt the butter. Add the onion and sauté until it's softened, about 2 minutes.

2. **Cook the spinach.** Stir in the spinach, vegetable broth, coconut cream, nutmeg, salt, and pepper and cook, giving it a stir from time to time, until the spinach is tender and the sauce thickens, about 15 minutes.

3. **Serve.** Put the creamed spinach in a bowl and serve.

Tip: This dish can also be baked if you don't want to spend time at the stove. After mixing all the ingredients together, transfer the mixture to a medium baking dish and bake, covered, in a 350°F oven for 15 minutes.

Swap: You can easily make this vegan if you want, by swapping in coconut oil for the butter.

Ditch the Dairy: Use 1 tablespoon of coconut oil instead of the butter.

PER SERVING
Macronutrients: Fat: 82%; Protein: 6%; Carbs: 12%
Calories: 85; Total fat: 8g; Total carbs: 3g; Fiber: 1g;
Net carbs: 2g; Sodium: 61mg; Protein: 1g

SIMPLE BUTTER-SAUTÉED VEGETABLES

SUPER QUICK

PREP TIME: 10 MINUTES | COOK TIME: 10 MINUTES
SERVES: 4

I'm willing to bet that before you started keto, you never sautéed your vegetables in butter because it's "not healthy." But now you know that it totally is, and that cooking them in chemicals (I'm looking at you, margarine) totally isn't. This recipe makes cooking veggies easy and fast, and it's good as a side for any kind of meat or fish. Feel free to swap in lower-carb vegetables here (like cauliflower, broccoli, and asparagus), though personally I love peppers. I also like to use different colored vegetables because they look really nice on the plate.

2 tablespoons
grass-fed butter

1 tablespoon
good-quality olive oil

2 teaspoons
minced garlic

2 zucchini, cut into
¼-inch rounds

1 red bell pepper, cut
into thick slices

1 yellow bell pepper,
cut into thick slices

Sea salt, for seasoning

Freshly ground black
pepper, for seasoning

1. **Cook the vegetables.** In a large skillet over medium-high heat, warm the butter and olive oil. Add the garlic and sauté it for 2 minutes. Add the zucchini and the red and yellow bell peppers to the skillet and sauté, stirring from time to time, for 7 minutes.

2. **Serve.** Season the vegetables with salt and pepper, spoon them into a bowl, and serve.

Tip: Sauté these vegetables right before you want to serve them because they do not hold up well to a long wait. This is a great dish to serve with grilled meat because you can easily make the vegetables and have them ready to serve by the time the meat is finished resting.

PER SERVING
Macronutrients: Fat: 82%; Protein: 3%; Carbs: 15%
Calories: 100; Total fat: 9g; Total carbs: 4g; Fiber: 1g;
Net carbs: 3g; Sodium: 67mg; Protein: 1g

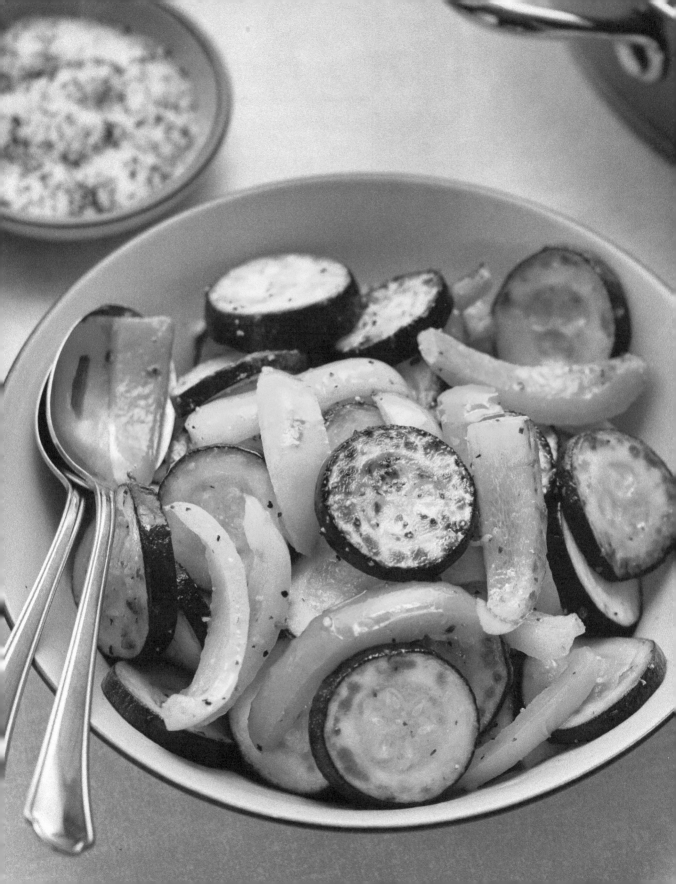

BUFFALO CAULIFLOWER BITES

SUPER QUICK

PREP TIME: 10 MINUTES | COOK TIME: 20 MINUTES

SERVES: 4

These bites are the perfect replacement for the deep-fried buffalo wings I used to eat—they're so good and so much healthier. Cauliflower soaks up whatever sauce or seasoning you cook it in, so it's a great, low-carb way to highlight the flavors of my spicy buffalo sauce. (If you're curious, the difference between plain hot sauce and buffalo sauce is adding butter.) So if you buy hot sauce or even buffalo sauce off the shelf, still add a couple tablespoons of butter for a better flavor and texture (and always make sure the sauce is sugar-free).

¾ cup hot sauce, divided

½ cup chicken stock

2 tablespoons grass-fed butter, melted

1 tablespoon coconut flour

1 head cauliflower, cut into small florets

1. **Preheat the oven.** Set the oven temperature to 450°F. Line a baking sheet with parchment paper.

2. **Prepare the sauce.** In a large bowl, whisk together the hot sauce, chicken stock, melted butter, and coconut flour until everything is well blended.

3. **Prepare the cauliflower.** Add the cauliflower florets to the sauce and stir to get them completely coated with sauce.

4. **Bake and serve.** Spread the cauliflower on the baking sheet and bake until it's tender, about 20 minutes. Put the cauliflower in a bowl and serve.

Tip: Dip the Buffalo Cauliflower Bites in blue cheese dressing for the complete taste experience.

Swap: Feel free to use this sauce on the chicken wings on page 72 instead of the orange-ginger sauce.

Ditch the Dairy: Use 2 tablespoons of duck fat instead of butter.

PER SERVING
Macronutrients: Fat: 69%; Protein: 11%; Carbs: 20%
Calories: 94; Total fat: 8g; Total carbs: 5g; Fiber: 2g;
Net carbs: 3g; Sodium: 1244mg; Protein: 3g

TENDER GRILLED ASPARAGUS SPEARS

SUPER QUICK

PREP TIME: 5 MINUTES | COOK TIME: 5 MINUTES
SERVES: 4

I love grilling vegetables because it's one of the easiest and tastiest ways to prepare them. When you're picking your asparagus, look for stalks that are about the width of a pencil and have tight heads and a consistent green color. I know that sounds a little nuts, but trust me, all that stuff makes a difference to the taste. If you've got a grill basket, this is the time to use it, otherwise you might lose some of the thinner stalks when they fall through the slats on your grill.

1 pound fresh asparagus spears, woody ends snapped off

2 tablespoons good-quality olive oil

Sea salt, for seasoning

Freshly ground black pepper, for seasoning

1. **Preheat the grill.** Set the grill to high heat.

2. **Prepare the asparagus.** In a medium bowl, toss the asparagus spears with the olive oil and season them with salt and pepper.

3. **Grill and serve.** Grill the asparagus until tender, 2 to 4 minutes. Arrange them on a platter and serve.

Tip: For a truly delicious dish, top the grilled asparagus with grated hardboiled egg and a generous drizzle of melted butter.

Swap: Red, yellow, or orange bell pepper, zucchini, and broccoli can all be prepared using this method with stellar results.

PER SERVING
Macronutrients: Fat: 74%; Protein: 7%; Carbs: 19%
Calories: 82; Total fat: 7g; Total carbs: 5g; Fiber: 2g;
Net carbs: 3g; Sodium: 27mg; Protein: 2g

SAUTÉED WILD MUSHROOMS WITH BACON

SUPER QUICK

PREP TIME: 10 MINUTES | COOK TIME: 15 MINUTES

SERVES: 4

When you feel like you've been eating the same green vegetables over and over, you can really switch things up with these mushrooms. They go perfectly with grilled meats, chicken, or fish, and they taste like something you'd get at a nice steakhouse. If you use different mushrooms, like portobello, oyster, cremini, white, and shiitake, it'll make for a nice-looking presentation and give you a good variety of textures. It's also totally fine to be lazy and just use one type, like white mushrooms. Just make sure to serve the mushrooms right away, because they're at their best when they're hot and the bacon is crackling.

6 strips uncured bacon, chopped

4 cups sliced wild mushrooms

2 teaspoons minced garlic

2 tablespoons chicken stock

1 tablespoon chopped fresh thyme

1. **Cook the bacon.** In a large skillet over medium-high heat, cook the bacon until it's crispy and cooked through, about 7 minutes.

2. **Cook the mushrooms.** Add the mushrooms and garlic and sauté until the mushrooms are tender, about 7 minutes.

3. **Deglaze the pan.** Add the chicken stock and stir to scrape up any browned bits in the bottom of the pan.

4. **Garnish and serve.** Put the mushrooms in a bowl, sprinkle them with the thyme, and serve.

Tip: If you are using portobello mushrooms, scoop out the black gills before slicing them so they don't discolor the rest of the dish.

PER SERVING
Macronutrients: Fat: 80%; Protein: 13%; Carbs: 7%
Calories: 214; Total fat: 19g; Total carbs: 4g; Fiber: 0g;
Net carbs: 4g; Sodium: 154mg; Protein: 7g

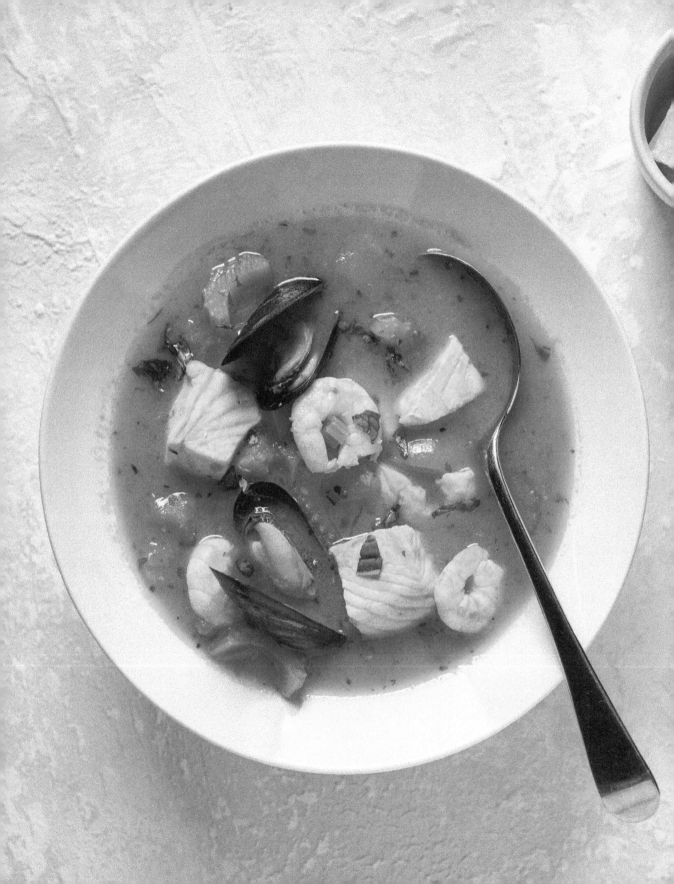

5

Soups and Salads

These soups and salads can be served as appetizers, but make no mistake, these can all be delicious, filling main courses, too. The soups are thick and hearty, and the salads have a great mix of healthy vegetables and proteins.

CHILI-INFUSED LAMB SOUP

SUPER QUICK

PREP TIME: 5 MINUTES | COOK TIME: 25 MINUTES

SERVES: 6

I grew up in a family of hunters. We had a house in upstate New York that served as a hunting house/getaway for my family to just be together in the outdoors. On the way there, my favorite thing to do in the wintertime was stop at small-town diners along the way and eat chili and local meat soups to warm us up. This soup always reminds me of those times growing up, and so it's become my favorite on a cold day. It warms me down to my toes and tastes amazing. Plus, chile peppers are really good for your metabolism. They also can help you eat less if your goal is to get fit because the nutrients in chiles reduce the hunger hormone (called ghrelin) produce by your body.

1 tablespoon coconut oil

¾ pound ground lamb

2 cups shredded cabbage

½ onion, chopped

2 teaspoons minced garlic

4 cups chicken broth

2 cups coconut milk

1½ tablespoons red chili paste or as much as you want

Zest and juice of 1 lime

1 cup shredded kale

1. **Cook the lamb.** In a medium stockpot over medium-high heat, warm the coconut oil. Add the lamb and cook it, stirring it often, until it has browned, about 6 minutes.

2. **Cook the vegetables.** Add the cabbage, onion, and garlic and sauté until they've softened, about 5 minutes.

3. **Simmer the soup.** Stir in the chicken broth, coconut milk, red chili paste, lime zest, and lime juice. Bring it to a boil, then reduce the heat to low and simmer until the cabbage is tender, about 10 minutes.

4. **Add the kale.** Stir in the kale and simmer the soup for 3 more minutes.

5. **Serve.** Spoon the soup into six bowls and serve.

Swap: For a hotter dish, swap the red chili paste for habanero or Scotch bonnet peppers. If you're using fresh peppers, wash your hands and equipment very well afterward to avoid burning yourself with the juices.

PER SERVING
Macronutrients: Fat: 74%; Protein: 20%; Carbs: 6%
Calories: 380; Total fat: 32g; Total carbs: 7g; Fiber: 1g;
Net carbs: 6g; Sodium: 290mg; Protein: 17g

NEW ENGLAND CLAM CHOWDER

PREP TIME: 10 MINUTES | COOK TIME: 30 MINUTES
SERVES: 8

I like to think of clam chowder like a heavyweight boxing champ—it's made restaurants and even entire regions of the country famous. Like most people, I love the stuff, but since the traditional recipe has potato chunks, it's not keto. Fortunately, I put together a potato-free recipe that comes out so creamy and rich you won't even miss 'em. Plus, you're getting a lot of nutritional benefits from the clams.

¼ pound uncured bacon, chopped

2 tablespoons grass-fed butter

½ onion, finely chopped

1 celery stalk, chopped

2 teaspoons minced garlic

2 tablespoons arrowroot

4 cups fish or chicken stock

1 teaspoon chopped fresh thyme

2 bay leaves

3 (6½-ounce) cans clams, drained

1½ cups heavy (whipping) cream

Sea salt, for seasoning

Freshly ground black pepper, for seasoning

2 tablespoons chopped fresh parsley

1. **Cook the bacon.** In a medium stockpot over medium-high heat, fry the bacon until it's crispy. Transfer the bacon with a slotted spoon to a plate and set it aside.

2. **Sauté the vegetables.** Melt the butter in the stockpot, add the onion, celery, and garlic and sauté them until they've softened, about 3 minutes. Whisk in the arrowroot and cook for 1 minute. Add the stock, thyme, and bay leaves and bring the soup to just before it boils. Then reduce the heat to medium-low and simmer until the soup thickens, about 10 minutes.

3. **Finish the soup.** Stir in the clams and cream and simmer the soup until it's heated through, about 5 minutes. Find and throw out the bay leaves.

4. **Serve.** Season the chowder with salt and pepper. Ladle it into bowls, garnish with the parsley, and crumbles of the bacon, then serve.

Tip: If you want to freeze this soup, make it through step 2 and let it cool to room temperature before putting it in an airtight container in the freezer. To reheat, let it thaw, add the clams and cream, and cook until it's heated through.

PER SERVING
Macronutrients: Fat: 65%; Protein: 25%; Carbs: 10%
Calories: 384; Total fat: 28g; Total carbs: 8g; Fiber: 2g;
Net carbs: 6g; Sodium: 231mg; Protein: 23g

CREAMY GREEK LEMON CHICKEN SOUP

FULL GUIDO

PREP TIME: 10 MINUTES | COOK TIME: 30 MINUTES

SERVES: 6

When my mom moved to this country from Italy, her first job was hosting and managing Greek diners. She worked at them for years, and I used to go to them a lot growing up, to visit her, and to eat the food. (I still do, don't worry!) This soup isn't exactly the traditional recipe like I used to get at those Greek restaurants, but it's definitely inspired by it. The (keto) problem with avgolemono soup is that it's low fat and contains orzo rice. This version is higher fat and obviously doesn't use rice. I like to make this soup when I'm having guests because it's got a complex and interesting taste that makes people think you worked over the stove for hours, but it's actually pretty simple to make. I use roasted chicken because it adds even more great flavor to the soup, but really any kind of cooked chicken would work.

½ cup grass-fed butter

½ onion, chopped

2 celery stalks, chopped

2 teaspoons minced garlic

¼ cup arrowroot

5 cups chicken stock

3 cups shredded cooked chicken

Zest and juice of 1 lemon

1 cup heavy (whipping) cream

Sea salt, for seasoning

Freshly ground black pepper, for seasoning

1 tablespoon chopped fresh oregano

1. **Sauté the vegetables.** In a medium stockpot over medium-high heat, melt the butter. Add the onion, celery, and garlic and sauté until they've softened, about 5 minutes.

2. **Make the soup base.** Add the arrowroot and whisk until it forms a paste. Whisk in the chicken stock.

3. **Thicken the soup.** Bring the soup to a boil, then reduce the heat to low and simmer, stirring it from time to time, until the soup thickens, about 15 minutes.

4. **Add the remaining ingredients.** Stir in the chicken, lemon zest, lemon juice, and cream and simmer until the chicken is heated through, about 10 minutes.

5. **Season and serve.** Season the soup with salt and pepper. Ladle the soup into bowls, garnish with the oregano, and serve it hot.

Tip: You can also use the "slurry" method to make the soup base. Whisk the arrowroot into ½ cup of the chicken stock and then whisk it into the soup rather than adding the arrowroot to the vegetables.

PER SERVING
Macronutrients: Fat: 65%; Protein: 25%; Carbs: 10%
Calories: 501; Total fat: 36g; Total carbs: 13g; Fiber: 3g;
Net carbs: 10g; Sodium: 339mg; Protein: 28g

CIOPPINO SEAFOOD SOUP

FULL GUIDO

PREP TIME: 10 MINUTES | COOK TIME: 30 MINUTES
SERVES: 6

Cioppino comes from the Italian name *ciuppin*, which is a seafood soup from Liguria, Italy. The cioppino seafood soup you might know, though, is actually a twist on that classic Italian recipe that started in San Francisco as a way to use up leftover fish in the 1800s. I guess I'm following that tradition, then, because this soup makes for good leftovers, too—on the second day, the flavor will be even better. This recipe has a lot of ingredients, but it's so tasty, I don't think you'll mind when you're slurping up a bowl of it.

2 tablespoons olive oil

½ onion, chopped

2 celery stalks, sliced

1 red bell pepper, chopped

1 tablespoon minced garlic

2 cups fish stock

1 (15-ounce) can coconut milk

1 cup crushed tomatoes

2 tablespoons tomato paste

1 tablespoon chopped fresh basil

2 teaspoons chopped fresh oregano

½ teaspoon sea salt

½ teaspoon freshly ground black pepper

ingredients continue on next page

1. **Sauté the vegetables.** In a large stockpot over medium-high heat, warm the olive oil. Add the onion, celery, red bell pepper, and garlic and sauté until they've softened, about 4 minutes.

2. **Make the soup base.** Stir in the fish stock, coconut milk, crushed tomatoes, tomato paste, basil, oregano, salt, pepper, and red pepper flakes. Bring the soup to a boil, then reduce the heat to low and simmer the soup for 10 minutes.

3. **Add the seafood.** Stir in the salmon and simmer until it goes opaque, about 5 minutes. Add the shrimp and simmer until they're almost cooked through, about 3 minutes. Add the mussels and let them simmer until they open, about 3 minutes. Throw out any mussels that don't open.

¼ teaspoon red pepper flakes

10 ounces salmon, cut into 1-inch pieces

½ pound shrimp, peeled and deveined

12 clams or mussels, cleaned and debearded but in the shell (see the Tip)

4. Serve. Ladle the soup into bowls and serve it hot.

Tip: Scrub the mussels very well so your broth isn't gritty, and pull out the tough "beard" sticking out of the shell. Wait until an hour before cooking to do this because debearding will kill the mussel.

PER SERVING
Macronutrients: Fat: 65%; Protein: 26%; Carbs: 9%
Calories: 377; Total fat: 29g; Total carbs: 9g; Fiber: 2g;
Net carbs: 7g; Sodium: 358mg; Protein: 24g

COCONUT SHRIMP SAFFRON SOUP

SUPER QUICK | FULL GUIDO

PREP TIME: 5 MINUTES | COOK TIME: 15 MINUTES

SERVES: 4

I'm a big fan of this soup because it shows that you can still eat exotic foods on keto. Here's something you probably never made before, and now you'll make it *and* it'll be keto-friendly. Saffron is really expensive because it comes from a crocus flower and it takes more than 5,000 flowers to produce one ounce of the stuff. But you only need a few strands of saffron to give the soup a deep color and flavor. You'll want to make this soup when you're having people over because it looks awesome and has a sophisticated taste. I like to serve it as a starter before a grilled chicken or beef dinner out on the patio.

1 tablespoon coconut oil

1 red bell pepper, chopped

2 teaspoons minced garlic

2 teaspoons grated fresh ginger

4 cups chicken stock

1 (15-ounce) can coconut milk

1 pound shrimp, peeled, deveined, and chopped

1 cup shredded kale

Juice of 1 lime

½ cup warm water

Pinch saffron threads

Sea salt, for seasoning

2 tablespoons chopped fresh cilantro

1. **Sauté the vegetables.** In a large saucepan over medium heat, warm the coconut oil. Add the red pepper, garlic, and ginger and sauté until they've softened, about 5 minutes.

2. **Simmer the soup.** Add the chicken stock and coconut milk and bring the soup to a boil, then reduce the heat to low and stir in the shrimp, kale, and lime juice. Simmer the soup until the shrimp is cooked through, about 5 minutes.

3. **Mix in the saffron.** While the soup is simmering, stir the saffron and the warm water together in a small bowl and let it sit for 5 minutes. Stir the saffron mixture into the soup when the shrimp is cooked, and simmer the soup for 3 minutes more.

4. **Season and serve.** Season with salt. Ladle the soup into bowls, garnish it with the cilantro, and serve it hot.

Tip: As mentioned above, there's a reason that saffron is expensive, so if you come across some that is cheap, take a close look to make sure it's the real deal. Take a look at the threads, and if the saffron is a uniform color on the whole strand (instead of having a lighter tip), it is probably not real saffron.

PER SERVING
Macronutrients: Fat: 65%; Protein: 23%; Carbs: 12%
Calories: 504; Total fat: 36g; Total carbs: 15g; Fiber: 3g;
Net carbs: 12g; Sodium: 334mg; Protein: 32g

LOADED SALAD BOWL

SUPER QUICK | FULL GUIDO

PREP TIME: 15 MINUTES

SERVES: 2

Lunch is usually the hardest meal for people to grasp on keto. Everyone is so used to eating sandwiches, bagels, wraps (anything you can hold in your hand, really). This dish can be your new sandwich . . . in a bowl . . . and you eat it with a fork. I usually make this when I want a meal that feels super healthy. Or sometimes just when I want to use up everything in my fridge! So yeah, feel free to substitute ingredients here based on what you like to eat or what you've got on hand. I like using arugula because it's from the same family as cauliflower and broccoli (and so offers the same health benefits), but it's got the slightest hint of bitterness that just makes it work in salads. If you like a peppery taste, look for older, darker leaves of arugula, and if you want it milder, go for younger, paler leaves.

4 cups arugula

2 tablespoons good-quality olive oil

Sea salt, for seasoning

Freshly ground black pepper, for seasoning

2 (4-ounce) grilled boneless chicken breasts, sliced

1 avocado, diced

1 tomato, cut into wedges

½ red onion, thinly sliced

2 ounces goat cheese

1. **Dress the salad.** In a medium bowl, toss the arugula with the olive oil and season it with salt and pepper.

2. **Assemble and serve.** Divide the arugula between two plates and top it with grilled chicken, avocado, tomato, red onion, and goat cheese. Serve the salad chilled or at room temperature.

Tip: If you need riper avocados than the ones in your kitchen, put them in a paper bag with other perishable items (tomatoes, avocados, or fruit if you are eating it in small amounts) and the ethylene gas given off by the other items will speed up the ripening process. In as little as 12 hours your avocado will be perfect.

PER SERVING

Macronutrients: Fat: 65%; Protein: 27%; Carbs: 8%

Calories: 278; Total fat: 19g; Total carbs: 6g; Fiber: 3g;

Net carbs: 3g; Sodium: 126mg; Protein: 21g

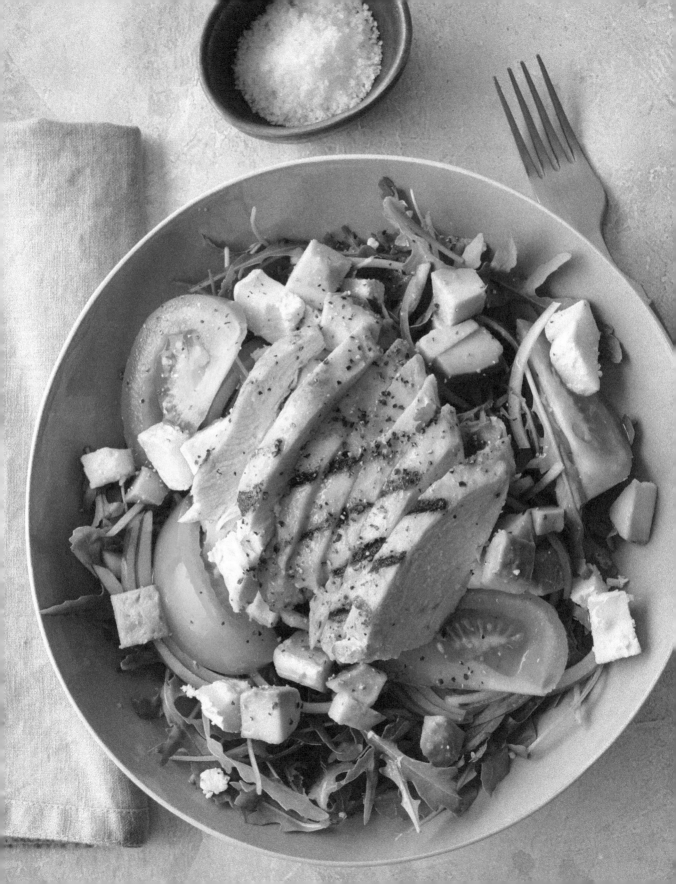

ANTIPASTO SALAD WITH SPIRALIZED ZUCCHINI

SUPER QUICK | FULL GUIDO

PREP TIME: 20 MINUTES

SERVES: 2

This is a salad but make no mistake, it's not an appetizer salad—this is a meal. It's hearty and packed with flavorful meats, marinated vegetables, and creamy cheese. This is the sort of colorful, delicious meal you'd want to serve for lunch on a warm summer day, sitting out on a shady patio. You'll need a spiralizer for this recipe, but it's a good thing to pick up anyway—it's a handy, inexpensive kitchen tool that you can use for zucchini and other vegetables to make salads like this or even to swap in for pasta noodles.

2 medium zucchini, spiralized

¼ cup Homemade Ranch Dressing (page 232)

2 ounces genoa salami, cut into thin strips

1 ounce pepperoni

1 ounce prosciutto, cut into thin strips

½ cup chopped artichoke hearts

¼ cup sliced Kalamata olives

¼ cup halved cherry tomatoes

Sea salt, for seasoning

Freshly ground black pepper, for seasoning

2 ounces mozzarella cheese, shredded

2 tablespoons chopped fresh parsley

1. **Mix the salad.** In a large bowl, toss together the zucchini noodles, ranch dressing, salami, pepperoni, prosciutto, artichokes, olives, and tomatoes.

2. **Season and serve.** Season the salad with salt and pepper. Divide the salad between two plates, garnish it with the mozzarella and parsley, and serve it immediately.

Swap: Try different meats—mortadella, bresaola, coppa, or sopressata—and sundried tomatoes, roasted red peppers, and mushrooms to create different delicious variations. These variations will change the nutrition data, but not enough to affect your macros for the day a whole lot.

PER SERVING

Macronutrients: Fat: 80%; Protein: 15%; Carbs: 5%
Calories: 492; Total fat: 44g; Total carbs: 8g; Fiber: 3g;
Net carbs: 5g; Sodium: 823mg; Protein: 18g

TUNA CHOPPED VEGETABLE LETTUCE CUPS

SUPER QUICK

PREP TIME: 15 MINUTES

SERVES: 2

The ingredients might look pretty humble, but don't be fooled—this recipe actually makes a really attractive salad with the mix of pale green and flecks of red and creamy white. This is an especially good recipe to make if you're going to be serving kids. I like to serve it to my little cousins. They love it because it feels familiar, and they can roll up the lettuce leaves and eat it with their hands. I use oil-packed tuna for the fat, so if you wind up using water-packed tuna, keep the keto macros right by adding in another fat source like shredded Cheddar.

2 (6-ounce) cans oil-packed tuna, drained and flaked

⅓ cup mayonnaise (I like to use Sir Kensington's or Primal Kitchen brands)

¼ cup finely chopped red bell pepper

1 celery stalk, finely chopped

1 scallion, chopped

2 tablespoons chopped olives

1 tablespoon small capers

4 large lettuce leaves

1 avocado, diced

1. **Mix the tuna salad.** In a medium bowl, mix together the tuna, mayonnaise, red bell pepper, celery, scallion, olives, and capers.

2. **Assemble the salad.** Spoon the tuna mixture into the lettuce leaves and top with the diced avocado.

3. **Serve.** Divide the filled lettuce leaves between two plates and serve.

Swap: Use the same amount of canned salmon or chopped chicken instead of tuna. You'll get equally nutritious, appealing results.

PER SERVING
Macronutrients: Fat: 58%; Protein: 32%; Carbs: 10%
Calories: 628; Total fat: 40g; Total carbs: 17g; Fiber: 8g;
Net carbs: 9g; Sodium: 453mg; Protein: 50g

SPINACH SALAD WITH SMOKED SALMON AND AVOCADO

SUPER QUICK

PREP TIME: 15 MINUTES

SERVES: 4

There was a time when smoked salmon was a hard-to-find luxury item, but now it's something you can find at most grocery stores. It's absolutely delicious and the coloring on the fish is gorgeous, plus it has lots of health benefits. When I'm making the salad dressing here, I usually will double or triple the recipe because it keeps for up to two weeks in the fridge—and it's so good I'll use it for pretty much all of my salads and marinades.

FOR THE DRESSING

½ cup good-quality olive oil

¼ cup white balsamic vinegar

¼ cup chopped fresh dill

1 teaspoon lemon zest

Sea salt, for seasoning

Freshly ground black pepper, for seasoning

FOR THE SALAD

6 cups fresh spinach, thoroughly washed and dried

1 pound smoked salmon, chopped

1 avocado, diced

½ red onion, chopped

½ cup crumbled goat cheese

¼ cup chopped pecans, divided

TO MAKE THE DRESSING

1. **Mix the dressing.** In a small bowl, whisk together the olive oil, vinegar, dill, and lemon zest.

2. **Season.** Season the dressing with salt and pepper and set it aside.

TO MAKE THE SALAD

1. **Mix the salad.** In a large bowl, toss together the spinach, salmon, avocado, and red onion until everything is well combined. Add the dressing to the salad and toss to coat all the ingredients with dressing.

2. **Assemble the salad.** Divide the salad evenly between four plates. Top each salad with goat cheese and pecans and serve.

Swap: Smoked trout is a good choice if you want a break from salmon. It's firmer and flakier, with a more delicate taste, and it contains almost all the same health benefits.

Ditch the Dairy: Leave out the goat cheese, and instead use ½ cup of chopped cooked bacon to increase the fat and protein.

PER SERVING
Macronutrients: Fat: 73%; Protein: 20%; Carbs: 7%
Calories: 540; Total fat: 45g; Total carbs: 9g; Fiber: 4g;
Net carbs: 5g; Sodium: 543mg; Protein: 26g

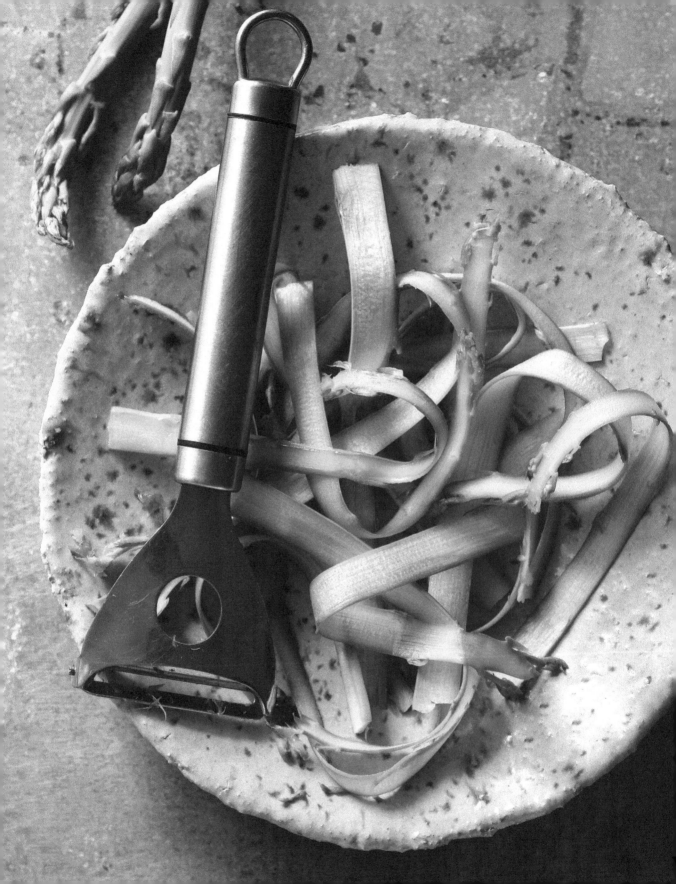

SHAVED ASPARAGUS SALAD WITH EGG

SUPER QUICK

PREP TIME: 20 MINUTES

SERVES: 4

This dish is great for a family get-together, a potluck, or even a fancy dinner. It all comes down to the preparation of the asparagus—it's unique, creative, and makes it taste so good. Plus, you're creating a gorgeous salad with dark green, white, and bright yellow. The best time to make this salad is the spring, when asparagus is in season.

FOR THE DRESSING

¼ cup good-quality olive oil

1½ tablespoons balsamic vinegar

½ teaspoon minced garlic

Sea salt, for seasoning

Freshly ground black pepper, for seasoning

FOR THE SALAD

½ pound asparagus stalks (about 20 medium), woody ends snapped off

4 hardboiled eggs, peeled and chopped

¼ cup chopped pecans

TO MAKE THE DRESSING

Mix the dressing. In a small bowl, stir together the olive oil, vinegar, and garlic. Season with salt and pepper and set it aside.

TO MAKE THE SALAD

1. **Prepare the asparagus.** Use a vegetable peeler to make long, thin asparagus ribbons, and put them in a large bowl.

2. **Mix the salad.** Add the eggs, pecans, and dressing to the asparagus and toss to combine the ingredients.

3. **Serve.** Divide the salad between four plates and serve.

Tip: If you want to make the salad ahead of time, don't add the eggs or pecans until just before serving and eating. Toss the asparagus ribbons with the dressing only.

PER SERVING

Macronutrients: Fat: 80%; Protein: 13%; Carbs: 7%
Calories: 254; Total fat: 23g; Total carbs: 5g; Fiber: 2g;
Net carbs: 3g; Sodium: 73mg; Protein: 8g

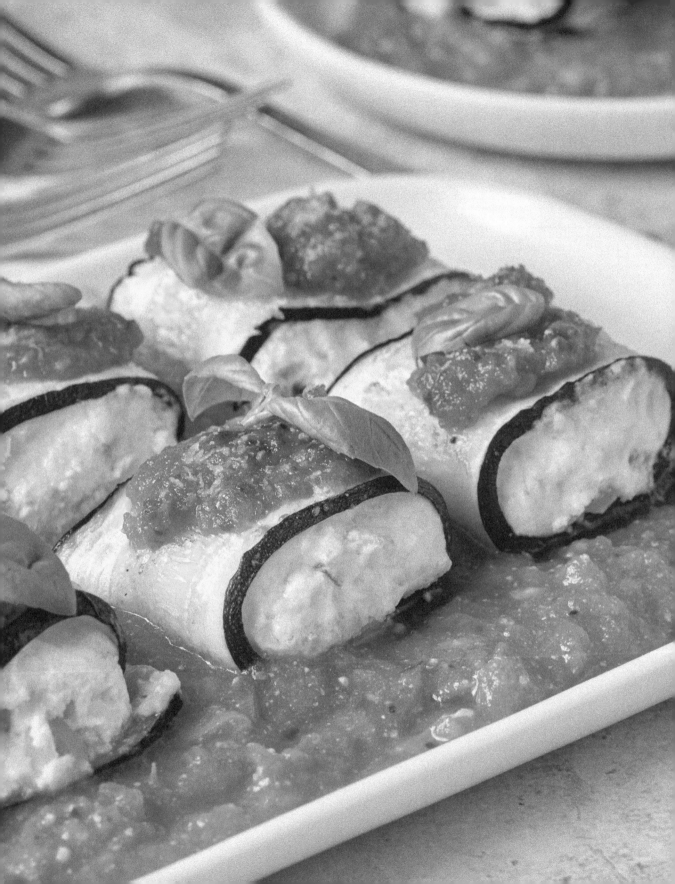

6

Vegetarian Mains

One of the biggest myths about keto is that it's all meat, all the time. People often think I just eat bacon and pepperoni all day, but I'm not always in the mood for meat, and that's when I use these vegetarian recipes. I also believe that fresh, organic veggies are the foundation of every healthy diet. People are surprised to realize that I have more in common with healthy vegetarians than I do with most of the population on the Standard American Diet because we both believe in eating real food that comes from the earth. My mom always served vegetables when I was growing up, so I make sure I have plenty of them on the table to this day.

CHEESY GARDEN VEGGIE CRUSTLESS QUICHE

SUPER QUICK

PREP TIME: 5 MINUTES | COOK TIME: 25 MINUTES

SERVES: 4

Apparently, quiches were invented in Germany as a peasant meal to use up a bunch of cheap, common ingredients. Later they became a fancy meal in France. With my recipe, I take it back to those roots—as a great way to make something tasty out of whatever you have in your fridge. Toss in arugula, bell peppers, cheeses, and, if you don't want to keep this vegetarian, some meat or whatever else you've got to switch up the recipe.

1 tablespoon grass-fed butter, divided

6 eggs

¾ cup heavy (whipping) cream

3 ounces goat cheese, divided

½ cup sliced mushrooms, chopped

1 scallion, white and green parts, chopped

1 cup shredded fresh spinach

10 cherry tomatoes, cut in half

1. **Preheat the oven.** Set the oven temperature to 350°F. Grease a 9-inch pie plate with ½ teaspoon of the butter and set it aside.

2. **Mix the quiche base.** In a medium bowl, whisk the eggs, cream, and 2 ounces of the cheese until it's all well blended. Set it aside.

3. **Sauté the vegetables.** In a small skillet over medium-high heat, melt the remaining butter. Add the mushrooms and scallion and sauté them until they've softened, about 2 minutes. Add the spinach and sauté until it's wilted, about 2 minutes.

4. **Assemble and bake.** Spread the vegetable mixture in the bottom of the pie plate and pour the egg-and-cream mixture over the vegetables. Scatter the cherry tomatoes and the remaining 1 ounce of goat cheese on top. Bake for 20 to 25 minutes until the quiche is cooked through, puffed, and lightly browned.

5. **Serve.** Cut the quiche into wedges and divide it between four plates. Serve it warm or cold.

Tip: You can bake this in muffin tins as well if handy, grab-and-go quiches work better for you. Grease the cups of a 6-cup muffin tin, divide the vegetable mixture between them, and pour in the egg mixture. Bake them for 12 to 15 minutes. This will not change the macros, but your calories will be 237 per "muffin."

PER SERVING
Macronutrients: Fat: 75%; Protein: 20%; Carbs: 5%
Calories: 355; Total fat: 30g; Total carbs: 5g; Fiber: 1g;
Net carbs: 4g; Sodium: 228mg; Protein: 18g

MEDITERRANEAN FILLING STUFFED PORTOBELLO MUSHROOMS

FULL GUIDO

PREP TIME: 10 MINUTES | COOK TIME: 35 MINUTES

SERVES: 4

Portobello mushrooms are a big staple of vegetarian cooking because they're filling, they're meaty, and they're the perfect container for any kind of filling. My Mediterranean filling just so happens to be one of the best. I use pecans in it because they're good for your heart, boost your metabolism, and can even help fight against cancer, plus they taste great and their texture works perfectly with the other ingredients. But if you don't like pecans or don't have any around, you can use other nuts instead.

4 large portobello
    mushroom caps

3 tablespoons
    good-quality olive
    oil, divided

1 cup chopped
    fresh spinach

1 red bell pepper,
    chopped

1 celery stalk, chopped

½ cup chopped sun-
    dried tomato

¼ onion, chopped

2 teaspoons
    minced garlic

1 teaspoon chopped
    fresh oregano

2 cups chopped pecans

¼ cup balsamic
    vinaigrette

Sea salt, for seasoning

Freshly ground black
    pepper, for seasoning

1. **Preheat the oven.** Set the oven temperature to 350°F. Line a baking sheet with parchment paper.

2. **Prepare the mushrooms.** Use a spoon to scoop the black gills out of the mushrooms. Massage 2 tablespoons of the olive oil all over the mushroom caps and place the mushrooms on the prepared baking sheet. Set them aside.

3. **Prepare the filling.** In a large skillet over medium-high heat, warm the remaining 1 tablespoon of olive oil. Add the spinach, red bell pepper, celery, sundried tomato, onion, garlic, and oregano and sauté until the vegetables are tender, about 10 minutes. Stir in the pecans and balsamic vinaigrette and season the mixture with salt and pepper.

4. **Assemble and bake.** Stuff the mushroom caps with the filling and bake for 20 to 25 minutes until they're tender and golden.

5. **Serve.** Place one stuffed mushroom on each of four plates and serve them hot.

Tip: Serve with a large mixed green salad or a bowl of creamy soup for a hearty meal.

PER SERVING
Macronutrients: Fat: 80%; Protein: 7%; Carbs: 13%
Calories: 595; Total fat: 56g; Total carbs: 18g; Fiber: 9g;
Net carbs: 9g; Sodium: 51mg; Protein: 10g

ZUCCHINI ROLL MANICOTTI

FULL GUIDO

PREP TIME: 15 MINUTES | COOK TIME: 30 MINUTES
SERVES: 4

I grew up eating pasta, so one of my big goals on keto has been to find a way to keep having the flavors and textures I love but without all the carbs. This zucchini roll manicotti is one of the best pasta substitute recipes I've come up with. When you eat a baked casserole like this, it'll take you right back to all of those boisterous family meals you had as a kid (if you came from a family like mine!). These rolls come out looking really nice, and you can even layer them up if you want a different look with the same flavors. The best part, though? You won't even miss the traditional pasta. I always say that the pasta itself is usually just the foundation you need to eat the real tasty stuff (the sauce and cheese), so if you can find a healthier, low-carb foundation (like this recipe), you will be set.

Olive oil cooking spray

4 zucchini

2 tablespoons
good-quality olive oil

1 red bell pepper, diced

½ onion, minced

2 teaspoons
minced garlic

1 cup goat cheese

1 cup shredded
mozzarella cheese

1 tablespoon chopped
fresh oregano

Sea salt, for seasoning

Freshly ground black
pepper, for seasoning

2 cups low-carb marinara
sauce, divided

½ cup grated
Parmesan cheese

1. **Preheat the oven.** Set the oven temperature to 375°F. Lightly grease a 9-by-13-inch baking dish with olive oil cooking spray.

2. **Prepare the zucchini.** Cut the zucchini lengthwise into ⅛-inch-thick slices and set them aside.

3. **Make the filling.** In a medium skillet over medium-high heat, warm the olive oil. Add the red bell pepper, onion, and garlic and sauté until they've softened, about 4 minutes. Remove the skillet from the heat and transfer the vegetables to a medium bowl. Stir the goat cheese, mozzarella, and oregano into the vegetables. Season it all with salt and pepper.

4. **Assemble the manicotti.** Spread 1 cup of the marinara sauce in the bottom of the baking dish. Lay a zucchini slice on a clean cutting board and place a couple tablespoons of

filling at one end. Roll the slice up and place it in the baking dish, seam-side down. Repeat with the remaining zucchini slices. Spoon the remaining sauce over the rolls and top with the Parmesan.

5. **Bake.** Bake the rolls for 30 to 35 minutes until the zucchini is tender and the cheese is golden.

6. **Serve.** Spoon the rolls onto four plates and serve them hot.

Tip: If you have time, you can lightly blanch the zucchini slices and drain them before rolling so that the casserole has less liquid in it from the juices and the slices roll easily. To blanch: Dunk the zucchini slices in boiling water. Leave them there for about 3 minutes, then remove them and run them under cold water or put them in a bowl filled with ice water for a few minutes to stop them from cooking any more.

PER SERVING
Macronutrients: Fat: 63%; Protein: 14%; Carbs: 23%
Calories: 342; Total fat: 24g; Total carbs: 14g; Fiber: 3g;
Net carbs: 11g; Sodium: 331mg; Protein: 20g

SPINACH ARTICHOKE STUFFED PEPPERS

SUPER QUICK | FULL GUIDO
PREP TIME: 10 MINUTES | COOK TIME: 20 MINUTES
SERVES: 4

Stuffed vegetables show up in most world cuisines, with different cultures scooping out everything from tomatoes to zucchini. These peppers are part of that tradition, but they go to a very decadent place. I'm talking peppers packed with melted cheeses and sour cream, so it's almost like you're eating classic spinach dip as a meal. I like to eat these with a simple mixed green salad and use balsamic vinaigrette or oil and vinegar as my dressing.

4 red bell peppers, halved and seeded

1 tablespoon good-quality olive oil, for drizzling

Sea salt, for seasoning

Freshly ground black pepper, for seasoning

2 cups finely chopped cauliflower

10 ounces chopped fresh spinach

2 cups chopped marinated artichoke hearts

1 cup cream cheese, softened

1½ cups shredded mozzarella cheese, divided

½ cup sour cream

2 tablespoons mayonnaise

2 teaspoons minced garlic

1. **Preheat the oven.** Set the oven temperature to 400°F. Line a baking sheet with parchment paper.

2. **Prepare the peppers.** Place the red bell peppers cut-side up on the baking sheet. Lightly grease them all over with the olive oil and season them with salt and pepper.

3. **Make the filling.** In a large bowl, mix together the cauliflower, spinach, artichoke hearts, cream cheese, ¾ cup of the mozzarella, and the sour cream, mayonnaise, and garlic.

4. **Stuff and bake.** Stuff the peppers with the filling and sprinkle with the remaining ¾ cup of mozzarella. Bake them for 20 to 25 minutes until the filling is heated through, bubbly, and lightly browned.

5. **Serve.** Place one stuffed pepper on each of four plates and serve them hot.

Swap: Use goat cheese instead of cream cheese and thick Greek-style yogurt instead of sour cream for a satisfying tangy flavor and velvety texture. This swap will change the macros to Fat: 62%; Protein: 26%; Carbs: 12%.

PER SERVING
Macronutrients: Fat: 72%; Protein: 16%; Carbs: 12%
Calories: 523; Total fat: 43g; Total carbs: 19g; Fiber: 7g;
Net carbs: 12g; Sodium: 355mg; Protein: 19g

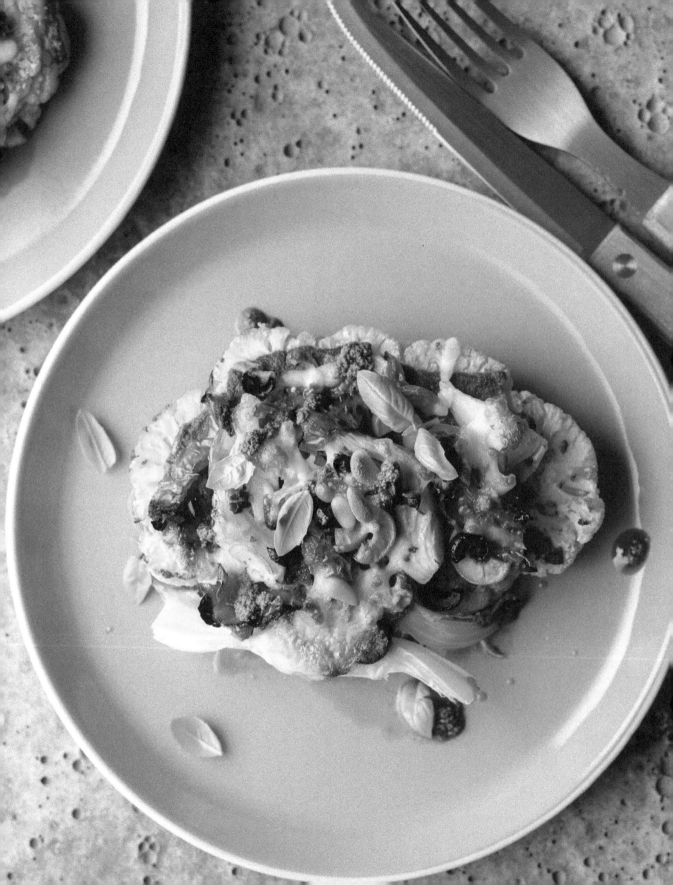

PESTO-GLAZED CAULIFLOWER STEAKS WITH FRESH BASIL AND MOZZARELLA

SUPER QUICK | FULL GUIDO
PREP TIME: 10 MINUTES | COOK TIME: 20 MINUTES
SERVES: 4

I like to eat real steak, so I'm just trying to help out my vegetarian friends with this recipe. Just kidding—this veggie steak dish is actually really good. My trick is to create the "steaks" by taking a large head of cauliflower and cutting thick enough slices that they stay together in one big slab. You can also experiment with the pesto here—like sometimes when I want to switch it up, I find sundried tomato pesto works really well with all the other ingredients.

Olive oil cooking spray

1 head cauliflower, cut into "steaks" about 1 inch thick

¼ cup Spinach Basil Pesto (page 224)

1 cup shredded mozzarella cheese

¼ cup chopped marinated artichoke hearts

¼ cup chopped sun-dried tomatoes

¼ cup sliced olives

2 tablespoons pine nuts

1. **Preheat the oven.** Set the oven temperature to 400°F. Lightly grease a baking sheet with olive oil cooking spray.

2. **Assemble the cauliflower steaks.** Place the cauliflower steaks in a single layer on the baking sheet and spread 1 tablespoon of pesto on each. Sprinkle with the mozzarella and top with the artichoke hearts, sundried tomatoes, olives, and pine nuts.

3. **Bake.** Bake the cauliflower for 20 minutes until the edges are crispy and the cheese is bubbly and melted.

4. **Serve.** Divide the cauliflower between four plates and serve it hot.

Tip: The center part of the cauliflower is the best for creating the steaks. There will be loose florets from the edges that won't stay together, which you can save and use in other recipes.

PER SERVING
Macronutrients: Fat: 65%; Protein: 18%; Carbs: 17%
Calories: 316; Total fat: 23g; Total carbs: 14g; Fiber: 6g;
Net carbs: 8g; Sodium: 465mg; Protein: 14g

ZUCCHINI PASTA WITH SPINACH, OLIVES, AND ASIAGO

SUPER QUICK | FULL GUIDO

PREP TIME: 10 MINUTES | COOK TIME: 10 MINUTES

SERVES: 4

You can't imagine how good this recipe looks until you're checking out the finished product in your kitchen. It's fresh, delicious, and absolutely stunning. Try throwing in a sprinkle of red pepper flakes or use a chili-infused olive oil for an extra kick. I usually make this zucchini pasta during the summer, because that's when zucchini, tomatoes, and basil are all in season and taste the best.

3 tablespoons good-quality olive oil

1 tablespoon grass-fed butter

1½ tablespoons minced garlic

1 cup packed fresh spinach

½ cup sliced black olives

½ cup halved cherry tomatoes

2 tablespoons chopped fresh basil

3 zucchini, spiralized

Sea salt, for seasoning

Freshly ground black pepper, for seasoning

½ cup shredded Asiago cheese

1. **Sauté the vegetables.** In a large skillet over medium-high heat, warm the olive oil and butter. Add the garlic and sauté until it's tender, about 2 minutes. Stir in the spinach, olives, tomatoes, and basil and sauté until the spinach is wilted, about 4 minutes. Stir in the zucchini noodles, toss to combine them with the sauce, and cook until the zucchini is tender, about 2 minutes.

2. **Serve.** Season with salt and pepper. Divide the mixture between four bowls and serve topped with the Asiago.

Tip: To save time, spiralize the zucchini ahead and store it in a sealed container in the fridge for up to three days, or buy it pre-spiralized.

PER SERVING
Macronutrients: Fat: 80%; Protein: 13%; Carbs: 7%
Calories: 199; Total fat: 18g; Total carbs: 4g; Fiber: 1g;
Net carbs: 3g; Sodium: 363mg; Protein: 6g

VEGETARIAN CHILI WITH AVOCADO AND SOUR CREAM

PREP TIME: 10 MINUTES | COOK TIME: 25 MINUTES
SERVES: 8

I've learned that chili is a big vegetarian staple—you won't find a vegetarian restaurant out there that doesn't have some kind of chili on the menu. But chili can be tough on keto because most of them go heavy on beans, and that just doesn't work on a keto diet. With my chili, there's no beans, just lots of really tasty vegetables and my secret ingredient: pecans. They add bulk, healthy fats, and protein, and oddly they feel a lot like ground beef when they're cooked.

2 tablespoons good-quality olive oil

½ onion, finely chopped

1 red bell pepper, diced

2 jalapeño peppers, chopped

1 tablespoon minced garlic

2 tablespoons chili powder

1 teaspoon ground cumin

4 cups canned diced tomatoes

2 cups pecans, chopped

1 cup sour cream

1 avocado, diced

2 tablespoons chopped fresh cilantro

1. **Sauté the vegetables.** In a large pot over medium-high heat, warm the olive oil. Add the onion, red bell pepper, jalapeño peppers, and garlic and sauté until they've softened, about 4 minutes. Stir in the chili powder and cumin, stirring to coat the vegetables with the spices.

2. **Cook the chili.** Stir in the tomatoes and pecans and bring the chili to a boil, then reduce the heat to low and simmer until the vegetables are soft and the flavors mellow, about 20 minutes.

3. **Serve.** Ladle the chili into bowls and serve it with the sour cream, avocado, and cilantro.

Tip: A handful of shredded Cheddar is a traditional topping for chili, so add a bit here if you want to lift the dish into classic status. A half-cup of shredded Cheddar will increase the fat by 2 grams and protein by 1 gram per portion.

PER SERVING
Macronutrients: Fat: 80%; Protein: 7%; Carbs: 13%
Calories: 332; Total fat: 32g; Total carbs: 11g; Fiber: 6g;
Net carbs: 5g; Sodium: 194mg; Protein: 5g

VEGETABLE VODKA SAUCE BAKE

FULL GUIDO

PREP TIME: 10 MINUTES | COOK TIME: 30 MINUTES

SERVES: 4

Growing up Italian, it's forbidden to eat traditional red sauce from anyone else besides your own family, but vodka sauce is the exception, and I actually prefer it when eating out at a restaurant or catered party. Maybe it's okay because vodka sauce isn't actually from Italy. It was created by Italian Americans as a mix of tomato sauce, Italian herbs, lots of heavy cream, and real vodka. The vodka is important because it brings out extra flavors and actually keeps the oil from separating. This definitely isn't an everyday kind of meal—it's so rich, you'll want to save it for special occasions. One note when you're making this is it may seem strange not to cook the mushrooms, but they'll get very tender just by baking in the sauce, and you don't want to overdo it.

3 tablespoons melted grass-fed butter, divided

4 cups mushrooms, halved

4 cups cooked cauliflower florets

1½ cups purchased vodka sauce (see Tip)

¾ cup heavy (whipping) cream

½ cup grated Asiago cheese

Sea salt, for seasoning

Freshly ground black pepper, for seasoning

1 cup shredded provolone cheese

2 tablespoons chopped fresh oregano

1. **Preheat the oven.** Set the oven temperature to 350°F and use 1 tablespoon of the melted butter to grease a 9-by-13-inch baking dish.

2. **Mix the vegetables.** In a large bowl, combine the mushrooms, cauliflower, vodka sauce, cream, Asiago, and the remaining 2 table-spoons of butter. Season the vegetables with salt and pepper.

3. **Bake.** Transfer the vegetable mixture to the baking dish and top it with the provolone cheese. Bake for 30 to 35 minutes until it's bubbly and heated through.

4. **Serve.** Divide the mixture between four plates and top with the oregano.

Tip: You can make your own vodka sauce if you have a favorite recipe, but there are many very good ones at the store that save time and money, which is why that's what I recommend here. Just be sure you're choosing one without any added sugar (or if you're making it from scratch, skip any recipe step that includes sugar).

PER SERVING
Macronutrients: Fat: 75%; Protein: 10%; Carbs: 15%
Calories: 537; Total fat: 45g; Total carbs: 14g; Fiber: 6g;
Net carbs: 8g; Sodium: 527mg; Protein: 19g

GREEK VEGETABLE BRIAM

FULL GUIDO

PREP TIME: 10 MINUTES | COOK TIME: 30 MINUTES

SERVES: 4

A *briam* is a Greek dish consisting of thinly sliced vegetables arranged over a bed of diced tomatoes and then roasted. It's something I used to eat at the Greek diners my mom worked at. My version isn't a totally traditional briam because I sauté the vegetables instead of roasting them, but it's still delicious. Greek food is part of the Mediterranean diet, which is similar to Italian food, and it also uses lots of fresh, healthy ingredients. When you're making this dish, don't forget the pumpkin seeds. They add a great crunch and a toasty flavor.

⅓ cup good-quality olive oil, divided

1 onion, thinly sliced

1 tablespoon minced garlic

¾ small eggplant, diced

2 zucchini, diced

2 cups chopped cauliflower

1 red bell pepper, diced

2 cups diced tomatoes

2 tablespoons chopped fresh parsley

2 tablespoons chopped fresh oregano

Sea salt, for seasoning

Freshly ground black pepper, for seasoning

1½ cups crumbled feta cheese

¼ cup pumpkin seeds

1. **Preheat the oven.** Set the oven to broil and lightly grease a 9-by-13-inch casserole dish with olive oil.

2. **Sauté the aromatics.** In a medium stockpot over medium heat, warm 3 tablespoons of the olive oil. Add the onion and garlic and sauté until they've softened, about 3 minutes.

3. **Sauté the vegetables.** Stir in the eggplant and cook for 5 minutes, stirring occasionally. Add the zucchini, cauliflower, and red bell pepper and cook for 5 minutes. Stir in the tomatoes, parsley, and oregano and cook, giving it a stir from time to time, until the vegetables are tender, about 10 minutes. Season it with salt and pepper.

4. **Broil.** Transfer the vegetable mixture to the casserole dish and top with the crumbled feta. Broil for about 4 minutes until the cheese is golden.

5. **Serve.** Divide the casserole between four plates and top it with the pumpkin seeds. Drizzle with the remaining olive oil.

Tip: This is a great dish to make ahead. Follow the recipe right up until it's ready to go under the broiler. Cover the casserole dish with aluminum foil and refrigerate for up to two days. To reheat, remove the foil and pop it in the oven at 375°F for a delicious meal in 20 minutes. Make sure you still broil it for a few minutes to create a golden top.

PER SERVING
Macronutrients: Fat: 70%; Protein: 11%; Carbs: 19%
Calories: 356; Total fat: 28g; Total carbs: 18g; Fiber: 7g;
Net carbs: 11g; Sodium: 467mg; Protein: 11g

CAULIFLOWER TIKKA MASALA

SUPER QUICK

PREP TIME: 10 MINUTES | COOK TIME: 20 MINUTES

SERVES: 4

If you've ever been to an Indian restaurant, you know the most common version of tikka masala is made with chicken. But I've found cauliflower soaks up the flavors of the sauce just as well. Swapping in cauliflower does complicate things a little, though. You're going to want to cook the cauliflower ahead of time; because the sauce is so thick, it's hard to cook a vegetable thoroughly in it. My version has a good amount of spice, but if you want it even spicier, add some cayenne pepper to the sauce.

FOR THE CAULIFLOWER

1 head cauliflower, cut into small florets

1 tablespoon coconut oil, melted

1 teaspoon ground cumin

½ teaspoon ground coriander

FOR THE SAUCE

2 tablespoons coconut oil

½ onion, chopped

1 tablespoon minced garlic

1 tablespoon grated ginger

2 tablespoons garam masala

1 tablespoon tomato paste

½ teaspoon salt

1 cup crushed tomatoes

1 cup heavy (whipping) cream

1 tablespoon chopped fresh cilantro

TO MAKE THE CAULIFLOWER

1. **Preheat the oven.** Set the oven temperature to 425°F. Line a baking sheet with aluminum foil.

2. **Prepare the cauliflower.** In a large bowl, toss the cauliflower with the coconut oil, cumin, and coriander. Spread the cauliflower on the baking sheet in a single layer and bake it for 20 minutes, until the cauliflower is tender.

TO MAKE THE SAUCE

1. **Sauté the vegetables.** While the cauliflower is baking, in a large skillet over medium-high heat, warm the coconut oil. Add the onion, garlic, and ginger and sauté until they've softened, about 3 minutes.

2. **Finish the sauce.** Stir in the garam masala, tomato paste, and salt until the vegetables are coated. Stir in the crushed tomatoes and bring to a boil, then reduce the heat to low and simmer the sauce for 10 minutes, stirring it often. Remove the skillet from the heat and stir in the cream and cilantro.

3. **Assemble and serve.** Add the cauliflower to the sauce, stirring to combine everything. Divide the mixture between four bowls and serve it hot.

Swap: If you don't need this dish to be vegetarian, try chunks of grilled chicken instead of cauliflower. This will increase the protein macro count for the dish, but obviously, it will no longer be vegetarian.

PER SERVING
Macronutrients: Fat: 75%; Protein: 8%; Carbs: 17%
Calories: 372; Total fat: 32g; Total carbs: 17g; Fiber: 7g;
Net carbs: 10g; Sodium: 346mg; Protein: 8g

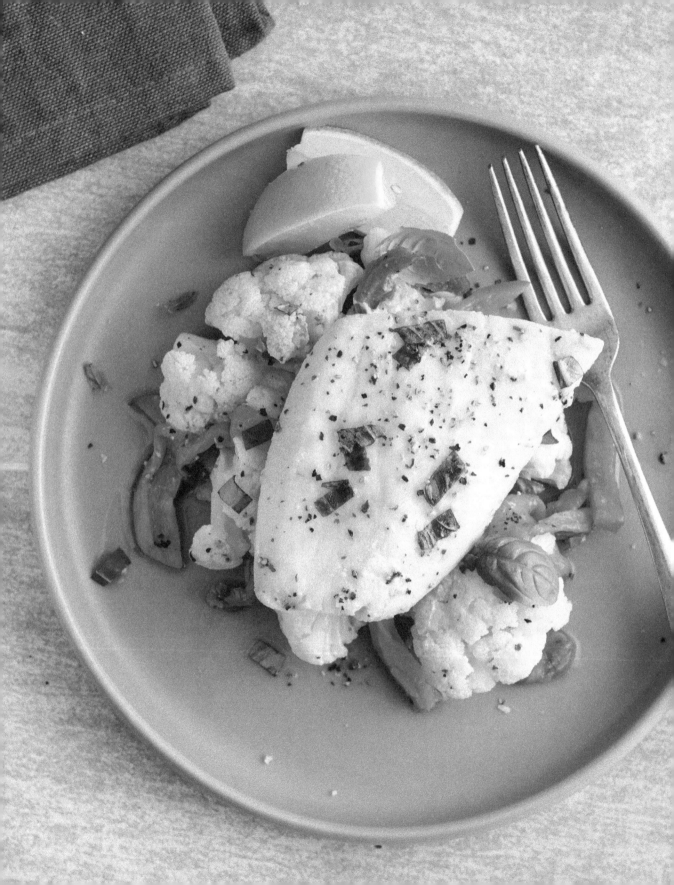

7

Seafood and Poultry

I try to vary up the types of meat I eat on keto, and that means lots of seafood and poultry dishes. These recipes are incredibly tasty, and they use the right ingredients to make sure you're still hitting your macros even with the leaner proteins. There's also something very primal about eating fish. My family is from a small beach town in Sicily called Sant'Agata di Militello where the majority of the diet is fresh-caught fish from the ocean, so I swear there's something in my DNA that makes my body crave seafood. When cooking seafood, aim to always get wild-caught fish—it's the healthiest and most delicious.

SIMPLE FLOUNDER IN BROWN BUTTER LEMON SAUCE

SUPER QUICK | FULL GUIDO

PREP TIME: 10 MINUTES | COOK TIME: 10 MINUTES

SERVES: 4

This presentation is humble, but it turns out spectacular, which just goes to show you that an amazing meal doesn't have to be complicated. Flounder is a flatfish that's high in protein and omega-3 fatty acids, and picking the right one is key. Get one that doesn't smell really "fishy." Also, look for a fish that has reddish gills and has a transparent slime on it, not a white slime. (I know that sounds gross, but the dish is tasty, I promise.)

FOR THE SAUCE

½ cup unsalted grass-fed butter, cut into pieces

Juice of 1 lemon

Sea salt, for seasoning

Freshly ground black pepper, for seasoning

FOR THE FISH

4 (4-ounce) boneless flounder fillets

Sea salt, for seasoning

Freshly ground black pepper, for seasoning

¼ cup almond flour

2 tablespoons good-quality olive oil

1 tablespoon chopped fresh parsley

TO MAKE THE SAUCE

1. **Brown the butter.** In a medium saucepan over medium heat, cook the butter, stirring it once in a while, until it is golden brown, about 4 minutes.

2. **Finish the sauce.** Remove the saucepan from the heat and stir in the lemon juice. Season the sauce with salt and pepper and set it aside.

TO MAKE THE FISH

1. **Season the fish.** Pat the fish fillets dry and season them lightly with salt and pepper. Spoon the almond flour onto a plate, then roll the fish fillets through the flour until they're lightly coated.

1. **Cook the fish.** In a large skillet over medium-high heat, warm the olive oil. Add the fish fillets and fry them until they're crispy and golden on both sides, 2 to 3 minutes per side.

2. **Serve.** Transfer the fish to a serving plate and drizzle with the sauce. Top with the parsley and serve it hot.

Swap: This simple, tasty dish can actually be made with any type of fish, from haddock to salmon to tilapia. The brown butter makes this one of the most delicious sauces for seafood. Period.

PER SERVING
Macronutrients: Fat: 74%; Protein: 22%; Carbs: 4%
Calories: 389; Total fat: 33g; Total carbs: 1g; Fiber: 0g;
Net carbs: 1g; Sodium: 256mg; Protein: 22g

GRILLED CALAMARI

SUPER QUICK | FULL GUIDO

PREP TIME: 10 MINUTES PLUS MARINATING TIME | COOK TIME: 5 MINUTES

SERVES: 4

I always get into the age-old debate with friends about how to pronounce "calamari." Italians from New York usually pronounce it like, "ga-la-mad," but my family is Italian and I'm first-generation American, so I always grew up pronouncing it the way they do, like "ca-la-ma-dee" (the real way!). However you say it, calamari is delicious. Some people don't like to eat the legs, but I don't mind them. The only thing that can really go wrong with calamari is if you overcook it—then it can get kind of rubbery and tough.

2 pounds calamari tubes and tentacles, cleaned

½ cup good-quality olive oil

Zest and juice of 2 lemons

2 tablespoons chopped fresh oregano

1 tablespoon minced garlic

¼ teaspoon sea salt

⅛ teaspoon freshly ground black pepper

1. **Prepare the calamari.** Score the top layer of the calamari tubes about 2 inches apart.

2. **Marinate the calamari.** In a large bowl, stir together the olive oil, lemon zest, lemon juice, oregano, garlic, salt, and pepper. Add the calamari and toss to coat it well, then place it in the refrigerator to marinate for at least 30 minutes and up to 1 hour.

3. **Grill the calamari.** Preheat a grill to high heat. Grill the calamari, turning once, for about 3 minutes total, until it's tender and lightly charred.

4. **Serve.** Divide the calamari between four plates and serve it hot.

Tip: If you are cleaning the calamari yourself, buy 25 to 50 percent more than the weight specified in the recipe because you will throw out up to half of it. So in this case, you'd need 2½ to 3 pounds uncleaned. Also, when you're cleaning it, make sure you get the cuttlebone out from inside the tube—it's the thing that looks and feels kinda like a transparent, flat straw.

Alternative method: This is a great recipe to use an air fryer with to make these into fried calamari. In that case, instead of grilling the calamari, air fry them at 375°F. Remove the squid from the marinade and drain. Spray the air fryer basket with olive oil cooking spray. Preheat the air fryer for 3 minutes. Add half of the calamari and cook for 8 to 10 minutes, shaking the basket once during cooking time, until the calamari are golden. Repeat with the remaining squid.

PER SERVING
Macronutrients: Fat: 60%; Protein: 33%; Carbs: 7%
Calories: 455; Total fat: 30g; Total carbs: 8g; Fiber: 1g;
Net carbs: 7g; Sodium: 101mg; Protein: 35g

SHRIMP SCAMPI

SUPER QUICK | FULL GUIDO
PREP TIME: 10 MINUTES | COOK TIME: 10 MINUTES
SERVES: 4

Scampi can mean two things: the type of seafood, and a specific dish made with butter and garlic. This is both. My recipe uses plain shrimp, but scampi should really be made with langoustines (that's the French word, I'm fancy) which are also called Dublin Bay Prawns. Adjust the garlic and herbs in this recipe to suit your taste—the amount of garlic I use is very generous.

3 tablespoons
grass-fed butter

2 tablespoons
good-quality olive oil

1 tablespoon
minced garlic

1 scallion, finely chopped

1 pound large shrimp
(31–35 pieces), peeled
and deveined

¼ cup white wine

Juice of 1 lemon

¼ teaspoon sea salt

⅛ teaspoon freshly
ground black pepper

2 tablespoons chopped
fresh parsley

1. **Sauté the aromatics.** In a large skillet over medium heat, warm the butter and olive oil. Add the garlic and scallion and sauté until they've softened, about 3 minutes.

2. **Cook the shrimp.** Add the shrimp to the skillet and sauté them until pink and just cooked through, 4 to 5 minutes. Transfer the shrimp to a plate with a slotted spoon.

3. **Finish the sauce.** Add the white wine and lemon juice to the skillet and bring to a boil, stirring it frequently. Remove the skillet from the heat and put the shrimp back into the skillet. Season them with the salt and pepper and toss to coat the shrimp.

4. **Serve.** Divide the shrimp between four plates and top with the parsley.

Tip: If you purchase frozen shrimp, thaw them in a covered colander set over a bowl in the refrigerator overnight, or place them in a sealed plastic bag and set it under cold running water for 10 minutes.

Ditch the Dairy: Use 3 tablespoons of coconut oil instead of butter.

PER SERVING
Macronutrients: Fat: 60%; Protein: 36%; Carbs: 4%
Calories: 269; Total Fat: 17g; Total Carbs: 3g; Fiber: 0g; Net Carbs: 3g; Sodium: 231mg; Protein: 23g

SOUVLAKI SPICED SALMON BOWLS

FULL GUIDO

PREP TIME: 10 MINUTES, PLUS MARINATING TIME | COOK TIME: 20 MINUTES

SERVES: 4

You've probably heard "souvlaki" used to talk about seasoned pork chunks on a skewer, but the herbs and spices used for that are just as delicious on salmon. The ingredients in the "bowl" part of this recipe aren't set in stone, so you can try artichoke hearts, arugula, or goat cheese, too. If you want an authentic Greek experience, use tzatziki on top instead of sour cream.

FOR THE SALMON

¼ cup good-quality olive oil

Juice of 1 lemon

2 tablespoons chopped fresh oregano

1 tablespoon minced garlic

1 tablespoon balsamic vinegar

1 tablespoon smoked sweet paprika

½ teaspoon sea salt

¼ teaspoon freshly ground black pepper

4 (4-ounce) salmon fillets

TO MAKE THE SALMON

1. **Marinate the fish.** In a medium bowl, stir together the olive oil, lemon juice, oregano, garlic, vinegar, paprika, salt, and pepper. Add the salmon and turn to coat it well with the marinade. Cover the bowl and let the salmon sit marinating for 15 to 20 minutes.

2. **Grill the fish.** Preheat the grill to medium-high heat and grill the fish until just cooked through, 4 to 5 minutes per side. Set the fish aside on a plate.

Swap: Chicken or grilled beef are wonderful options instead of salmon. This will lower the fat and protein in both cases—especially the chicken—by 11 grams fat and 1 gram protein.

FOR THE BOWLS

2 tablespoons good-quality olive oil

1 red bell pepper, cut into strips

1 yellow bell pepper, cut into strips

1 zucchini, cut into ½-inch strips lengthwise

1 cucumber, diced

1 large tomato, chopped

½ cup sliced Kalamata olives

6 ounces feta cheese, crumbled

½ cup sour cream

TO MAKE THE BOWLS

1. **Grill the vegetables.** In a medium bowl, toss together the oil, red and yellow bell peppers, and zucchini. Grill the vegetables, turning once, until they're lightly charred and soft, about 3 minutes per side.

2. **Assemble and serve.** Divide the grilled vegetables between four bowls. Top each bowl with cucumber, tomato, olives, feta cheese, and the sour cream. Place one salmon fillet on top of each bowl and serve immediately.

Tip: Tzatziki is easy to make from scratch. In a large bowl, mix together 1 cup of plain Greek yogurt, 1 large grated cucumber (with all the liquid squeezed out), 3 tablespoons of chopped fresh dill, 2 tablespoons of freshly squeezed lemon juice, and 1 teaspoon of minced garlic. Store in the refrigerator for up to one week.

PER SERVING

Macronutrients: Fat: 70%; Protein: 23%; Carbs: 7%
Calories: 553; Total fat: 44g; Total carbs: 10g; Fiber: 3g;
Net carbs: 7g; Sodium: 531mg; Protein: 30g

PROSCIUTTO-WRAPPED HADDOCK

SUPER QUICK | FULL GUIDO
PREP TIME: 10 MINUTES | COOK TIME: 15 MINUTES
SERVES: 4

You're going to be surprised how complex the flavors are in this dish, since it seems pretty basic and it's super easy to prepare. You can get garlic-infused olive oil in pretty much every grocery store, or you can make it yourself with lightly crushed garlic cloves. When you're wrapping the prosciutto, make sure you don't have any gaps—overlap the slices if they're smaller widths.

4 (4-ounce) haddock fillets, about 1 inch thick

Sea salt, for seasoning

Freshly ground black pepper, for seasoning

4 slices prosciutto (2 ounces)

3 tablespoons garlic-infused olive oil

Juice and zest of 1 lemon

1. **Preheat the oven.** Set the oven temperature to 350°F. Line a baking sheet with parchment paper.

2. **Prepare the fish.** Pat the fish dry with paper towels and season it lightly on both sides with salt and pepper. Wrap the prosciutto around the fish tightly but carefully so it doesn't rip.

3. **Bake the fish.** Place the fish on the baking sheet and drizzle it with the olive oil. Bake for 15 to 17 minutes until the fish flakes easily with a fork.

4. **Serve.** Divide the fish between four plates and top with the lemon zest and a drizzle of lemon juice.

Tip: Get your prosciutto sliced fresh at the deli for the best texture, and always look for Italian-imported products with a "DOP" symbol on the packaging. This means the prosciutto is regulated and the quality is guaranteed.

PER SERVING
Macronutrients: Fat: 60%; Protein: 2%; Carbs: 38%
Calories: 282; Total fat: 18g; Total carbs: 1g; Fiber: 0g;
Net carbs: 1g; Sodium: 76mg; Protein: 29g

GRILLED SALMON WITH CAPONATA

FULL GUIDO

PREP TIME: 15 MINUTES | COOK TIME: 20 MINUTES

SERVES: 4

Salmon is the perfect fish for grilling, since it's got a firm texture and it's nice and oily. Also it will "release" from the grill when it's ready to be turned, so don't try and turn it until you can slide your spatula under it easily. Be careful not to overcook the fish or it can get dry. A sign that you're close to overcooking is when you see white beads on the surface and sides.

¼ cup good-quality olive oil, divided

1 onion, chopped

2 celery stalks, chopped

1 tablespoon minced garlic

2 tomatoes, chopped

½ cup chopped marinated artichoke hearts

¼ cup pitted green olives, chopped

¼ cup cider vinegar

2 tablespoons white wine

2 tablespoons chopped pecans

4 (4-ounce) salmon fillets

Freshly ground black pepper, for seasoning

2 tablespoons chopped fresh basil

1. **Make the caponata.** In a large skillet over medium heat, warm 3 tablespoons of the olive oil. Add the onion, celery, and garlic, and sauté until they've softened, about 4 minutes. Stir in the tomatoes, artichoke hearts, olives, vinegar, white wine, and pecans. Bring the mixture to a boil, then reduce the heat to low and simmer until the liquid has reduced, 6 to 7 minutes. Remove the skillet from the heat and set it aside.

2. **Grill the fish.** Preheat a grill to medium-high heat. Pat the fish dry with paper towels and rub it with the remaining 1 tablespoon of olive oil and season lightly with black pepper. Grill the salmon, turning once, until it is just cooked through, about 8 minutes total.

3. **Serve.** Divide the salmon between four plates, top with a generous scoop of the caponata, and serve immediately with fresh basil.

Tip: The caponata can be made ahead, cooled completely, and stored in the refrigerator in a sealed container for 4 to 5 days.

PER SERVING

Macronutrients: Fat: 65%; Protein: 28%; Carbs: 7%
Calories: 348; Total fat: 25g; Total carbs: 7g; Fiber: 3g;
Net carbs: 4g; Sodium: 128mg; Protein: 24g

SWEET CRAB CAKES

SUPER QUICK

PREP TIME: 15 MINUTES, PLUS CHILLING TIME | COOK TIME: 10 MINUTES

SERVES: 4

My crab cakes are tender and citrusy, which makes them perfect plain, but you can enhance them with salsas or sauces (like my aioli recipe on page 230). You can also make these crab cakes ahead of time and freeze them on baking sheets, then transfer them to sealable plastic bags. When you're ready to make them, take out the number you need, thaw them in the fridge, and fry them up—and they'll still taste amazing.

1 pound cooked lump crabmeat, drained and picked over

¼ cup shredded unsweetened coconut

1 tablespoon Dijon mustard

1 scallion, finely chopped

¼ cup minced red bell pepper

1 egg, lightly beaten

1 teaspoon lemon zest

Pinch cayenne pepper

3 tablespoons coconut flour

3 tablespoons coconut oil

¼ cup Classic Aioli (page 230)

1. **Make the crab cakes.** In a medium bowl, mix together the crab, coconut, mustard, scallion, red bell pepper, egg, lemon zest, and cayenne until it holds together. (If the mixture doesn't hold together when pressed, mix in 1 tablespoon of almond flour.) Form the mixture into eight equal patties about ¾ inch thick.

2. **Chill.** Place the patties on a plate, cover the plate with plastic wrap, and chill them in the refrigerator for at least 1 hour and up to 12 hours.

3. **Coat the patties.** Spread the coconut flour on a plate. Dip each patty in the flour until it's lightly coated.

4. **Cook.** In a large skillet over medium heat, warm the coconut oil. Fry the crab-cake patties, turning them once, until they're golden and cooked through, about 5 minutes per side.

5. **Serve.** Place two crab cakes on each of four plates and serve with the aioli.

Tip: Don't stress about using fresh crab meat still in the legs and claws—great quality crab can be found in cans or frozen. Just avoid imitation products or these succulent cakes will not be the same!

Alternative method: This is a great recipe to use an air fryer with to give your crab cakes some crunch. In that case, instead of cooking the patties, air fry them at 350°F. Spray the air fryer basket with olive oil cooking spray and preheat for 3 minutes. Add the crab cakes to the basket, four at a time, in a single layer. Air fry for 5 minutes; carefully turn over each crab cake, and air fry for 5 to 6 minutes longer until golden. Repeat with the remaining four crab cakes.

PER SERVING
Macronutrients: Fat: 60%; Protein: 30% Carbs: 10%
Calories: 370; Total fat: 24g; Total carbs: 12g; Fiber: 6g;
Net carbs: 6g; Sodium: 652mg; Protein: 26g

HERBED COCONUT MILK STEAMED MUSSELS

SUPER QUICK

PREP TIME: 10 MINUTES | COOK TIME: 15 MINUTES

SERVES: 4

Mussels are my favorite food to eat on Christmas Eve when my family celebrates the seven fishes. This dish is so fragrant, it'll remind you of your own family gathering, or maybe just of going to a fancy restaurant, but it's still ridiculously easy to prepare. Mussels are available in most grocery stores, so they're not a difficult ingredient to come by. My favorites are the blue ones that are in season and available in the winter and spring. Store your mussels loosely wrapped in the fridge, so they can breathe, and cook them the same day if possible.

2 tablespoons coconut oil

½ sweet onion, chopped

2 teaspoons minced garlic

1 teaspoon grated fresh ginger

½ teaspoon turmeric

1 cup coconut milk

Juice of 1 lime

1½ pounds fresh mussels, scrubbed and debearded

1 scallion, finely chopped

2 tablespoons chopped fresh cilantro

1 tablespoon chopped fresh thyme

1. **Sauté the aromatics.** In a large skillet, warm the coconut oil. Add the onion, garlic, ginger, and turmeric and sauté until they've softened, about 3 minutes.

2. **Add the liquid.** Stir in the coconut milk and lime juice and bring the mixture to a boil.

3. **Steam the mussels.** Add the mussels to the skillet, cover, and steam until the shells are open, about 10 minutes. Take the skillet off the heat and throw out any unopened mussels.

4. **Add the herbs.** Stir in the scallion, cilantro, and thyme.

5. **Serve.** Divide the mussels and the sauce between four bowls and serve them immediately.

Tip: Take the time to sort through your mussels before using them in this recipe. Throw away any chipped or broken shells and any which are already open because that means they're dead. If you are unsure, tap any open shells—living mussels will close up tight.

PER SERVING
Macronutrients: Fat: 63%; Protein: 26%; Carbs: 11%
Calories: 319; Total fat: 23g; Total carbs: 8g; Fiber: 2g;
Net carbs: 6g; Sodium: 395mg; Protein: 23g

BASIL HALIBUT RED PEPPER PACKETS

SUPER QUICK | FULL GUIDO
PREP TIME: 10 MINUTES | COOK TIME: 20 MINUTES
SERVES: 4

So you might be wondering why I say you should cook your fish all folded up in packets. It's because those packets keep all the juices and seasonings together so you don't lose a single delicious drop. Halibut is a perfect fish for this traditional cooking method, which is called *en papillote* in France or *al cartoccio* in Italian. Halibut flesh is firm and falls away in juicy chunks instead of flaking, which is what you want. The other ingredients like the roasted red pepper and sundried tomatoes can be replaced by just about anything, like spinach, or olives.

2 cups cauliflower florets

1 cup roasted red pepper strips

½ cup sliced sun-dried tomatoes

4 (4-ounce) halibut fillets

¼ cup chopped fresh basil

Juice of 1 lemon

¼ cup good-quality olive oil

Sea salt, for seasoning

Freshly ground black pepper, for seasoning

1. **Preheat the oven.** Set the oven temperature to 400°F. Cut four (12-inch) square pieces of aluminum foil. Have a baking sheet ready.

2. **Make the packets.** Divide the cauliflower, red pepper strips, and sundried tomato between the four pieces of foil, placing the vegetables in the middle of each piece. Top each pile with 1 halibut fillet, and top each fillet with equal amounts of the basil, lemon juice, and olive oil. Fold and crimp the foil to form sealed packets of fish and vegetables and place them on the baking sheet.

3. **Bake.** Bake the packets for about 20 minutes, until the fish flakes with a fork. Be careful of the steam when you open the packet!

4. **Serve.** Transfer the vegetables and halibut to four plates, season with salt and pepper, and serve immediately.

Swap: If you want to copy professional chefs, try parchment paper folded in a similar manner to aluminum foil. Simply tuck the folded ends under the packets so they don't open up while cooking.

PER SERVING
Macronutrients: Fat: 55%; Protein: 35%; Carbs: 10%
Calories: 294; Total fat: 18g; Total carbs: 8g; Fiber: 3g;
Net carbs: 5g; Sodium: 114mg; Protein: 25g

BAKED CHICKEN CAPRESE

FULL GUIDO

PREP TIME: 15 MINUTES | COOK TIME: 40 MINUTES

SERVES: 4

Did you know that in Italy, "caprese" really just means a dish? In the US, we usually use it to mean a salad with mozzarella, tomatoes, and basil. No matter where you're from, you'll love this caprese. Try to use fresh mozzarella whenever you can because it's got a soft, moist texture and a fantastic milky flavor. Also, fresh mozzarella has a firm texture that shreds well, and it melts beautifully without hardening up.

4 (4-ounce) boneless chicken breasts

Sea salt, for seasoning

Freshly ground black pepper, for seasoning

¼ cup extra-virgin olive oil, divided

1 tablespoon minced garlic

1 (28-ounce) can sodium-free diced tomatoes

2 tablespoons chopped fresh basil

Pinch red pepper flakes

4 ounces shredded mozzarella cheese

1. **Preheat the oven.** Set the oven temperature to 400°F.

2. **Brown the chicken.** Pat the chicken breasts dry and season them lightly all over with salt and pepper. In a large oven-safe skillet over medium-high heat, warm 2 tablespoons of the olive oil. Brown the chicken on all sides, about 6 minutes in total. Transfer the chicken to a plate and set it aside.

3. **Make the sauce.** Add the remaining 2 tablespoons of olive oil and the garlic to the skillet and sauté until the garlic has softened, about 2 minutes. Stir in the tomatoes, basil, and red pepper flakes and cook for 5 minutes.

4. **Bake the chicken.** Return the chicken breasts to the skillet, spooning sauce over them, and sprinkle with the shredded mozzarella. Cover the skillet and bake for 25 minutes or until the chicken is cooked through.

5. **Serve.** Divide the chicken breasts between four plates, making sure to include the sauce, and serve immediately.

Swap: This is a very simple sauce with a rich tomato flavor. Fresh tomatoes are a good choice if you have nice ones from your garden or heirloom produce from the farmers' market.

PER SERVING
Macronutrients: Fat: 65%; Protein: 28%; Carbs: 7%
Calories: 432; Total fat: 32g; Total carbs: 9g; Fiber: 3g;
Net carbs: 6g; Sodium: 257mg; Protein: 29g

CHICKEN ROLLATINI WITH RICOTTA, PROSCIUTTO, AND SPINACH

FULL GUIDO
PREP TIME: 15 MINUTES | COOK TIME: 35 MINUTES
SERVES: 4

You might be surprised how professional this chicken rollatini looks when it's cooked and served. To make the presentation even more spectacular, let the rolls rest for 10 minutes and then cut them in half on the plates to serve. The filling in this dish has a really nice green, pink, and white pinwheel inside. And if you don't have prosciutto handy, you can swap in Parma ham or even regular ham.

4 (3-ounce) boneless skinless chicken breasts, pounded to about ⅓ inch thick

4 ounces ricotta cheese

4 slices prosciutto (4 ounces)

1 cup fresh spinach

½ cup almond flour

½ cup grated Parmesan cheese

2 eggs, beaten

¼ cup good-quality olive oil

1. **Preheat the oven.** Set the oven temperature to 400°F.

2. **Prepare the chicken.** Pat the chicken breasts dry with paper towels. Spread ¼ of the ricotta in the middle of each breast. Place the prosciutto over the ricotta and ¼ cup of the spinach on the prosciutto. Fold the long edges of the chicken breast over the filling, then roll the chicken breast up to enclose the filling. Place the rolls seam-side down on your work surface.

3. **Bread the chicken.** On a plate, stir together the almond flour and Parmesan and set it next to the beaten eggs. Carefully dip a chicken roll in the egg, then roll it in the almond-flour mixture until it is completely covered. Set the rolls seam-side down on your work surface. Repeat with the other rolls.

4. **Brown the rolls.** In a medium skillet over medium heat, warm the olive oil. Place the rolls seam-side down in the skillet and brown them on all sides, turning them carefully, about 10 minutes in total. Transfer the rolls, seam-side down, to a 9-by-9-inch baking dish.

5. **Bake.** Bake the chicken rolls for 25 minutes, or until they're cooked through.

6. **Serve.** Place one chicken roll on each of four plates and serve them immediately.

Tip: Ricotta cheese comes in many types, so look for whole-milk varieties so the fat content is higher. Also take a look at the label because ricotta can have added sugar.

PER SERVING
Macronutrients: Fat: 64%; Protein: 34%; Carbs: 2%
Calories: 438; Total fat: 30g; Total carbs: 2g; Fiber: 0g;
Net carbs: 2g; Sodium: 722mg; Protein: 40g

CHICKEN SCARPARIELLO WITH SPICY SAUSAGE

FULL GUIDO

PREP TIME: 10 MINUTES | COOK TIME: 45 MINUTES

SERVES: 6

Scarpariello means "shoemaker" in Italian and it describes a dish that could be made relatively quickly by Neapolitan shoemakers at the end of the day or during lunch. In Italy, some of these recipes include tomatoes, but in the American version, it's usually chicken, sausage, vinegar, onions, and peppers. This version uses dry white wine in place of vinegar, but you can use the same quantity of red wine vinegar instead.

1 pound boneless chicken thighs

Sea salt, for seasoning

Freshly ground black pepper, for seasoning

3 tablespoons good-quality olive oil, divided

½ pound Italian sausage (sweet or hot)

1 tablespoon minced garlic

1 pimiento, chopped

¼ cup dry white wine

1 cup chicken stock

2 tablespoons chopped fresh parsley

1. **Preheat the oven.** Set the oven temperature to 425°F.

2. **Brown the chicken and sausage.** Pat the chicken thighs dry with paper towels and season them lightly with salt and pepper. In a large oven-safe skillet over medium-high heat, warm 2 tablespoons of the olive oil. Add the chicken thighs and sausage to the skillet and brown them on all sides, turning them carefully, about 10 minutes.

3. **Bake the chicken and sausage.** Place the skillet in the oven and bake for 25 minutes or until the chicken is cooked through. Take the skillet out of the oven, transfer the chicken and sausage to a plate, and put the skillet over medium heat on the stovetop.

4. **Make the sauce.** Warm the remaining 1 tablespoon of olive oil, add the garlic and pimiento, and sauté for 3 minutes. Add the white wine and deglaze the skillet by using a spoon to scrape up any browned bits from the bottom of the skillet. Pour in the chicken stock and

bring it to a boil, then reduce the heat to low and simmer until the sauce reduces by about half, about 6 minutes.

5. **Finish and serve.** Return the chicken and sausage to the skillet, toss it to coat it with the sauce, and serve it topped with the parsley.

Swap: You can use a red bell pepper instead of a pimiento, but since pimientos (also called cherry peppers) are a mild chile pepper with a bit of heat, add a pinch of red pepper flakes to the bell pepper for a similar flavor.

PER SERVING
Macronutrients: Fat: 74%; Protein: 22%; Carbs: 4%
Calories: 370; Total fat: 30g; Total carbs: 3g; Fiber: 0g;
Net carbs: 3g; Sodium: 314mg; Protein: 19g

ALMOND CHICKEN CUTLETS

SUPER QUICK | FULL GUIDO

PREP TIME: 10 MINUTES | COOK TIME: 15 MINUTES

SERVES: 4

When I was young, my mom would make chicken cutlets and I would pick out only the thin, crispy ones to eat and leave all the big thick ones on my plate. So my mom started just making tiny, thin, crispy cutlets that were similar to chicken strips or popcorn chicken. I still prefer to make my cutlets this way today. The key is to make sure you pound the chicken very thin without tearing the meat so the cutlets are very crispy when they're done. In this keto-fied version, the nutty, sweet flavor of the almonds does wonders, and you won't miss the bread crumbs.

2 eggs

½ teaspoon garlic powder

1 cup almond flour

1 tablespoon chopped fresh oregano

4 (4-ounce) bone-less skinless chicken breasts, pounded to about ¼ inch thick

¼ cup good-quality olive oil

2 tablespoons grass-fed butter

1. **Bread the chicken.** Whisk together the eggs and garlic powder in a medium bowl and set it aside. Stir together the almond flour and oregano on a plate and set the plate next to the egg mixture. Pat the chicken breasts dry with paper towels and dip them into the egg mixture. Shake off any excess egg and roll the chicken in the almond flour until they're coated.

2. **Fry the chicken.** In a large skillet over medium-high heat, warm the olive oil and butter. Add the breaded chicken breasts and fry them, turning them once, until they're cooked through, very crispy, and golden brown, 14 to 16 minutes in total.

3. **Serve.** Place one cutlet on each of four plates and serve them immediately.

Tip: These cutlets are delicious as is, but they can also be the base of a traditional chicken Parmesan dish by adding sugar-free tomato sauce and a sprinkling of mozzarella. This will add additional carbs and a couple grams of fat to the dish.

Swap: This recipe would also be delicious with pork pounded flat the same way, but that would be called schnitzel instead.

Alternative method: This is a great recipe for the air fryer. Instead of frying the chicken cutlets on the stove, cook them in the air fryer at 360°F. Spray the basket with olive oil cooking spray. Preheat the air fryer for 3 minutes. Place the cutlets in the basket in a single layer. Air fry for 6 minutes, then flip each cutlet over, and cook for 3 to 4 minutes longer or until the chicken reaches 165°F.

Ditch the Dairy: Use 2 tablespoons of coconut oil instead of butter to increase the fat and protein in this dish.

PER SERVING
Macronutrients: Fat: 65%; Protein: 34%; Carbs: 1%
Calories: 328; Total fat: 23g; Total carbs: 0g; Fiber: 0g;
Net carbs: 0g; Sodium: 75mg; Protein: 28g

SLOW COOKER CHICKEN THIGHS WITH SUNDRIED TOMATOES

FULL GUIDO

PREP TIME: 10 MINUTES | COOK TIME: 10 MINUTES PLUS SLOW COOKER TIME
SERVES: 4

I could've called this recipe "double tomato chicken," but then you wouldn't envision the extra rich sweetness you'll get from the sundried tomatoes. Back in the day, sundried tomatoes were actually dried in the sun after they were sprinkled with salt to preserve them, but now most of them are produced in factories instead. So if you want that authentic old school flavor, dry your own quartered plum tomatoes in a single layer on a baking sheet in a 200°F oven overnight. Your tomatoes will have an intense flavor and they'll be slightly juicier.

¼ cup olive oil, divided

4 (4-ounce) boneless chicken thighs

Sea salt, for seasoning

Freshly ground black pepper, for seasoning

1 (28-ounce) can sodium-free diced tomatoes

½ cup chicken stock

4 ounces julienned oil-packed sundried tomatoes

2 tablespoons minced garlic

2 tablespoons dried oregano

Pinch red pepper flakes

2 tablespoons chopped fresh parsley

1. **Grease the slow cooker.** Coat the bowl of the slow cooker with 1 tablespoon of the olive oil.

2. **Brown the chicken.** Pat the chicken thighs dry with paper towels and season them lightly with salt and pepper. In a large skillet over medium-high heat, warm the remaining 3 tablespoons of olive oil. Add the chicken thighs and brown them, turning them once, about 10 minutes in total.

3. **Cook in the slow cooker.** Put the tomatoes, chicken stock, sundried tomatoes, garlic, oregano, and red pepper flakes into the slow cooker and stir to combine the ingredients. Add the chicken, making sure it is covered by the sauce, place the lid on the slow cooker, and cook it on high heat for 4 to 6 hours or on low heat for 6 to 8 hours.

4. **Serve.** Divide the chicken thighs and sauce between four bowls and top with the parsley.

Tip: If you are short on time, prepare the recipe the same way, but instead of putting all the ingredients in the slow cooker, put them in a baking dish, cover the dish with aluminum foil, and cook it for 1½ hours in a 375°F oven.

PER SERVING
Macronutrients: Fat: 70%; Protein: 20%; Carbs: 10%
Calories: 468; Total fat: 36g; Total carbs: 14g; Fiber: 7g;
Net carbs: 7g; Sodium: 213mg; Protein: 24g

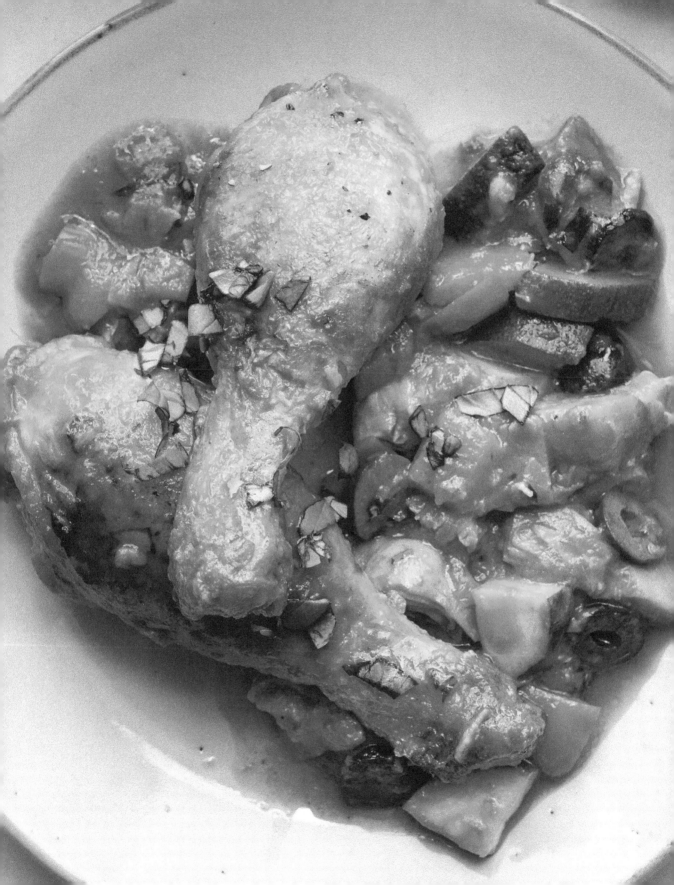

BRAISED CHICKEN LEGS WITH OLIVES AND ARTICHOKES

FULL GUIDO

PREP TIME: 15 MINUTES | COOK TIME: 45 MINUTES

SERVES: 4

There are two steps to braising in order to create succulent chicken: browning it and then cooking it in a sauce or liquid until it's tender. The browning step is crucial because chicken skin won't gain much color simmering gently in a sauce, and it won't look appealing, either. Browning adds texture, color, and flavor to the meat, which definitely improves the dish.

4 chicken legs

Sea salt, for seasoning

Freshly ground black pepper, for seasoning

¼ cup olive oil, divided

1 onion, chopped

1 red bell pepper, chopped

1 zucchini, chopped

2 tablespoons minced garlic

2 cups tomato sauce

1 cup chicken broth

1 cup chopped artichoke hearts

1 teaspoon smoked paprika

½ cup sliced Kalamata olives

2 tablespoons chopped fresh basil

1. **Brown the chicken.** Pat the chicken legs dry with a paper towel and season them lightly with salt and pepper. In a large skillet over medium-high heat, warm 2 tablespoons of the olive oil. Add the chicken legs and brown them, turning them once, about 10 minutes in total. Transfer them to a plate and set it aside.

2. **Sauté the vegetables.** Warm the remaining 2 tablespoons of olive oil in the skillet. Add the onion, red bell pepper, zucchini, and garlic and sauté until they've softened, about 5 minutes.

3. **Make the sauce.** Stir in the tomato sauce, chicken broth, artichoke hearts, and smoked paprika and bring it to a boil.

CONTINUED ▶

4. **Braise the chicken.** Reduce the heat to low and return the chicken and any accumulated juices on the plate to the skillet. Cover the skillet and simmer until the chicken is cooked through, 28 to 30 minutes. Remove the skillet from the heat and stir in the olives.

5. **Serve.** Divide the chicken between four plates and top with the chopped basil.

Swap: If you are "chickened" out, use 4 (5-ounce) pork chops instead of the chicken legs. Braise them for about 15 minutes more than the chicken legs, depending on how thick the chops are, to reach a 145°F internal temperature. This change in protein will not change the macros significantly if your pork chops weigh about 4 ounces each.

PER SERVING
Macronutrients: Fat: 65%; Protein: 27%; Carbs: 8%
Calories: 456; Total fat: 33g; Total carbs: 11g; Fiber: 4g;
Net carbs: 7g; Sodium: 281mg; Protein: 29g

SLOW COOKER CHICKEN CACCIATORE

FULL GUIDO

PREP TIME: 15 MINUTES | COOK TIME: 10 MINUTES PLUS SLOW COOKER TIME
SERVES: 4

Cacciatore comes from the Italian word for hunter, and usually includes sautéed and slow-cooked meat like chicken, rabbit, or veal combined with mushrooms, tomatoes, herbs, onions, and wine. This recipe is perfect for a slow cooker, spending hours just simmering in that delicious sauce to make your flavorful masterpiece. You can serve it plain, but I like to serve it over zucchini noodles or spaghetti sauce.

¼ cup good-quality olive oil

4 (4-ounce) boneless chicken breasts, each cut into three pieces

1 onion, chopped

2 celery stalks, chopped

1 cup sliced mushrooms

2 tablespoons minced garlic

1 (28-ounce) can sodium-free diced tomatoes

½ cup red wine

½ cup tomato paste

1 tablespoon dried basil

1 teaspoon dried oregano

⅛ teaspoon red pepper flakes

1. **Brown the chicken.** In a skillet over medium-high heat, warm the olive oil. Add the chicken breasts and brown them, turning them once, about 10 minutes in total.

2. **Cook in the slow cooker.** Place the chicken in the slow cooker and stir in the onion, celery, mushrooms, garlic, tomatoes, red wine, tomato paste, basil, oregano, and red pepper flakes. Cook it on high for 3 to 4 hours or on low for 6 to 8 hours, until the chicken is fully cooked and tender.

3. **Serve.** Divide the chicken and sauce between four bowls and serve it immediately.

Swap: Boneless chicken thighs are absolutely amazing in this recipe instead of breasts because they are juicier, generally. Don't get thighs with bones; it will be hard to find all the little bones after the meat is cooked.

PER SERVING
Macronutrients: Fat: 60%; Protein: 28%; Carbs: 12%
Calories: 383; Total fat: 26g; Total carbs: 11g; Fiber: 4g;
Net carbs: 7g; Sodium: 116mg; Protein: 26g

CHEESY CHICKEN SUNDRIED TOMATO PACKETS

FULL GUIDO

PREP TIME: 15 MINUTES | COOK TIME: 40 MINUTES

SERVES: 4

This dish is just downright pretty. It's golden and it oozes delicious cheese. If you have access to chicken supremes, which are chicken breasts with the small wing drumstick attached, use those here for an even better look. You can stuff the chicken ahead of time and store covered in the refrigerator for a day until you're ready to cook them.

1 cup goat cheese

½ cup chopped oil-packed sundried tomatoes

1 teaspoon minced garlic

½ teaspoon dried basil

½ teaspoon dried oregano

4 (4-ounce) boneless chicken breasts

Sea salt, for seasoning

Freshly ground black pepper, for seasoning

3 tablespoons olive oil

1. **Preheat the oven.** Set the oven temperature to 375°F.

2. **Prepare the filling.** In a medium bowl, stir together the goat cheese, sundried tomatoes, garlic, basil, and oregano until everything is well blended.

3. **Stuff the chicken.** Make a horizontal slice in the middle of each chicken breast to make a pocket, making sure not to cut through the sides or ends. Spoon one-quarter of the filling into each breast, folding the skin and chicken meat over the slit to form packets. Secure the packets with a toothpick. Lightly season the breasts with salt and pepper.

4. **Brown the chicken.** In a large oven-safe skillet over medium heat, warm the olive oil. Add the breasts and sear them, turning them once, until they are golden, about 8 minutes in total.

5. **Bake the chicken.** Place the skillet in the oven and bake the chicken for 30 minutes or until it's cooked through.

6. **Serve.** Remove the toothpicks. Divide the chicken between four plates and serve them immediately.

Swap: Replace the goat cheese with the same amount of cream cheese and add 1 teaspoon of fresh lemon juice to get a creamier filling with the same tangy flavor.

PER SERVING
Macronutrients: Fat: 68%; Protein: 29%; Carbs: 3%
Calories: 388; Total fat: 29g; Total carbs: 4g; Fiber: 1g;
Net carbs: 3g; Sodium: 210mg; Protein: 28g

TUSCAN CHICKEN SAUTÉ

FULL GUIDO

PREP TIME: 10 MINUTES | COOK TIME: 35 MINUTES

SERVES: 4

Tuscany is a region in central Italy that's famous for its beautiful artwork, vineyards, and *cucina povera* (or "poor cooking")—food created with inexpensive ingredients in large quantities, like this dish. The olive oil, garlic, fresh greens, and herbs make a wonderful base here. I add cream, which I'll admit isn't a traditional Tuscan preparation, but it adds richness and texture to this simple dish.

1 pound boneless chicken breasts, each cut into three pieces

Sea salt, for seasoning

Freshly ground black pepper, for seasoning

3 tablespoons olive oil

1 tablespoon minced garlic

¾ cup chicken stock

1 teaspoon dried oregano

½ teaspoon dried basil

½ cup heavy (whipping) cream

½ cup shredded Asiago cheese

1 cup fresh spinach

¼ cup sliced Kalamata olives

1. **Prepare the chicken.** Pat the chicken breasts dry and lightly season them with salt and pepper.

2. **Sauté the chicken.** In a large skillet over medium-high heat, warm the olive oil. Add the chicken and sauté until it is golden brown and just cooked through, about 15 minutes in total. Transfer the chicken to a plate and set it aside.

3. **Make the sauce.** Add the garlic to the skillet and sauté until it's softened, about 2 minutes. Stir in the chicken stock, oregano, and basil, scraping up any browned bits in the skillet. Bring to a boil, then reduce the heat to low and simmer until the sauce is reduced by about one-quarter, about 10 minutes.

4. **Finish the dish.** Stir in the cream and Asiago and simmer, stirring the sauce frequently, until it has thickened, about 5 minutes. Return the chicken to the skillet along with any accumulated juices. Stir in the spinach and olives and simmer until the spinach is wilted, about 2 minutes.

5. **Serve.** Divide the chicken and sauce between four plates and serve it immediately.

Swap: Swiss chard or kale are good alternatives to spinach if you enjoy a slightly earthier taste than spinach. Use tender baby kale rather than large leaves because the bigger ones can be tough and fibrous.

PER SERVING
Macronutrients: Fat: 70%; Protein: 26%; Carbs: 4%
Calories: 483; Total fat: 38g; Total carbs: 5g; Fiber: 1g;
Net carbs: 3g; Sodium: 332mg; Protein: 31g

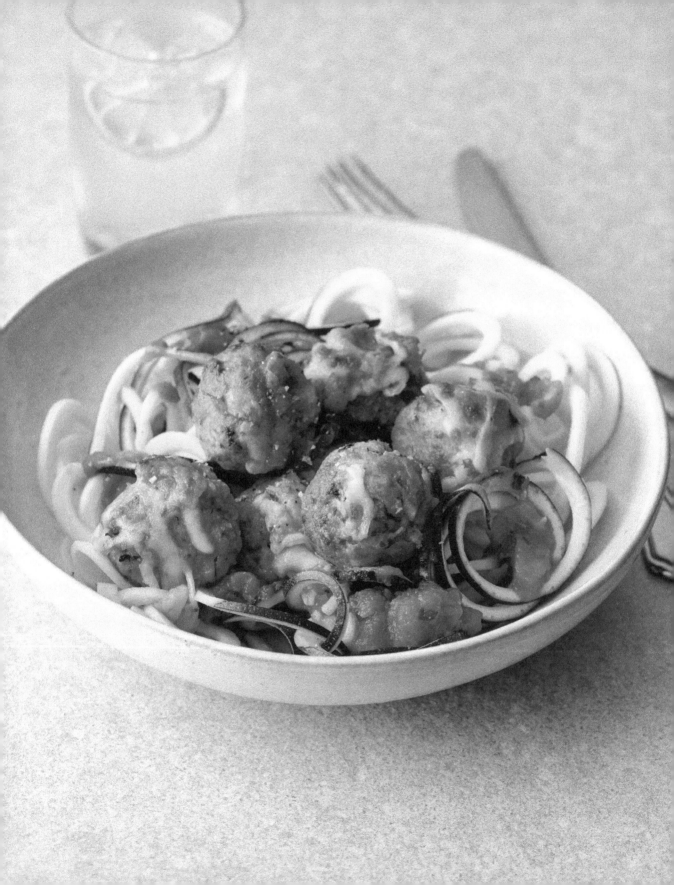

8

Pork and Beef

As I've mentioned earlier in the book, I am a big fan of steak. In fact, I could throw a steak on the grill every night and be happy. But it's good to change things up, so in this chapter I'm giving you lots of different beef and pork recipes, made different ways. Hopefully these many ways of cooking and eating delicious, fatty meats will mean that you'll never get bored.

PORK CHOPS WITH PECAN CRUST

PREP TIME: 10 MINUTES | COOK TIME: 25 MINUTES
SERVES: 4

The pecan crust on these pork chops hits perfect keto macros. Pecans are high in heart-healthy unsaturated fat and disease-fighting antioxidants—in fact, they've got the highest level of antioxidants of any tree nut. If you don't like cheese or you feel like you've eaten enough for the day, you can make the crust without the Parmesan.

2 eggs, lightly beaten

2 tablespoons
    coconut milk

1½ cups finely
    chopped pecans

¼ cup Parmesan cheese

4 (4-ounce) pork
    loin chops, about
    ½ inch thick

Sea salt, for seasoning

Freshly ground black
    pepper, for seasoning

2 tablespoons
    good-quality olive oil

1. **Prepare the pork chops.** Stir together the eggs and coconut milk in a small bowl. On a small plate, mix the pecans and Parmesan together and set the plate beside the egg mixture. Pat the pork chops dry and season them lightly with salt and pepper. Dip the pork chops first in the egg mixture, letting the excess run off, then roll them through the pecan mixture so they're coated. Set them aside on a plate.

2. **Fry the pork.** In a large skillet over medium heat, warm the olive oil. Fry the pork chops in a single layer, turning them several times, until they're cooked through and golden, 10 to 12 minutes per side.

3. **Serve.** Divide the pork chops between four plates and serve them immediately.

Swap: The pecans can be replaced by almonds or walnuts for a less sweet preparation. The trick is to chop the nuts finely so they get good coverage on the chops.

PER SERVING
Macronutrients: Fat: 72%; Protein: 23%; Carbs: 5%
Calories: 567; Total fat: 48g; Total carbs: 6g; Fiber: 4g;
Net carbs: 2g; Sodium: 373mg; Protein: 33g

CILANTRO GARLIC PORK CHOPS

SUPER QUICK

PREP TIME: 10 MINUTES, PLUS MARINATING TIME | COOK TIME: 15 MINUTES
SERVES: 4

Cilantro can definitely be an acquired taste, and here it's a very distinctive addition. But if you don't like it, try using the same amount of parsley or a couple tablespoons of chopped oregano. I recommend cilantro because it's pungent and it's available year-round. If you can't find something good and fresh, pick up the tubes of puréed herbs in the produce section and use about two tablespoons.

1 pound boneless
  center-cut pork chops,
  pounded to ¼ inch thick

Sea salt, for seasoning

Freshly ground black
  pepper, for seasoning

¼ cup good-quality
  olive oil, divided

¼ cup finely chopped
  fresh cilantro

1 tablespoon
  minced garlic

Juice of 1 lime

1. **Marinate the pork.** Pat the pork chops dry and season them lightly with salt and pepper. Place them in a large bowl, add 2 tablespoons of the olive oil, and the cilantro, garlic, and lime juice. Toss to coat the chops. Cover the bowl and marinate the chops at room temperature for 30 minutes.

2. **Cook the pork.** In a large skillet over medium-high heat, warm the remaining 2 tablespoons of olive oil. Add the pork chops in a single layer and fry them, turning them once, until they're just cooked through and still juicy, 6 to 7 minutes per side.

3. **Serve.** Divide the chops between four plates and serve them immediately.

Tip: Although marinating is considered a good way to tenderize meat, be careful when using an acidic marinade like this one for longer than 30 minutes because the meat will actually toughen.

PER SERVING
Macronutrients: Fat: 60%; Protein: 37%; Carbs: 3%
Calories: 249; Total fat: 16g; Total carbs: 2g; Fiber: 0g;
Net carbs: 2g; Sodium: 261mg; Protein: 25g

SPINACH FETA STUFFED PORK

FULL GUIDO

PREP TIME: 15 MINUTES | COOK TIME: 30 MINUTES

SERVES: 4

There's a popular Greek appetizer called spanakopita that inspired my ingredients here: spinach, feta, and olives. Yum. Kalamata olives are only found on the Peloponnese peninsula in southern Greece, and they're usually large and black or brown. You could substitute any other black olives in this recipe, but Kalamata olives have a truly wonderful texture and flavor that's worth the extra cost.

4 ounces crumbled feta cheese

¾ cup chopped frozen spinach, thawed and liquid squeezed out

3 tablespoons chopped Kalamata olives

4 (4-ounce) center pork chops, 2 inches thick

Sea salt, for seasoning

Freshly ground black pepper, for seasoning

3 tablespoons good-quality olive oil

1. **Preheat the oven.** Set the oven temperature to 400°F.

2. **Make the filling.** In a small bowl, mix together the feta, spinach, and olives until everything is well combined.

3. **Stuff the pork chops.** Make a horizontal slit in the side of each chop to create a pocket, making sure you don't cut all the way through. Stuff the filling equally between the chops and secure the slits with toothpicks. Lightly season the stuffed chops with salt and pepper.

4. **Brown the chops.** In a large oven-safe skillet over medium-high heat, warm the olive oil. Add the chops and sear them until they're browned all over, about 10 minutes in total.

5. **Roast the chops.** Place the skillet in the oven and roast the chops for 20 minutes or until they're cooked through.

6. **Serve.** Let the meat rest for 10 minutes and then remove the toothpicks. Divide the pork chops between four plates and serve them immediately.

Swap: If you want to use fresh spinach (about 8 cups), blanch it for a few minutes and squeeze out as much liquid as possible so that the filling is not runny. To blanch: Dunk the spinach in boiling water. Leave it there for about 3 minutes, then remove it and run it under cold water or put it in a bowl filled with ice water for a few minutes to stop it from cooking any more.

PER SERVING
Macronutrients: Fat: 62%; Protein: 34%; Carbs: 4%
Calories: 342; Total fat: 24g; Total carbs: 3g; Fiber: 1g;
Net carbs: 2g; Sodium: 572mg; Protein: 28g

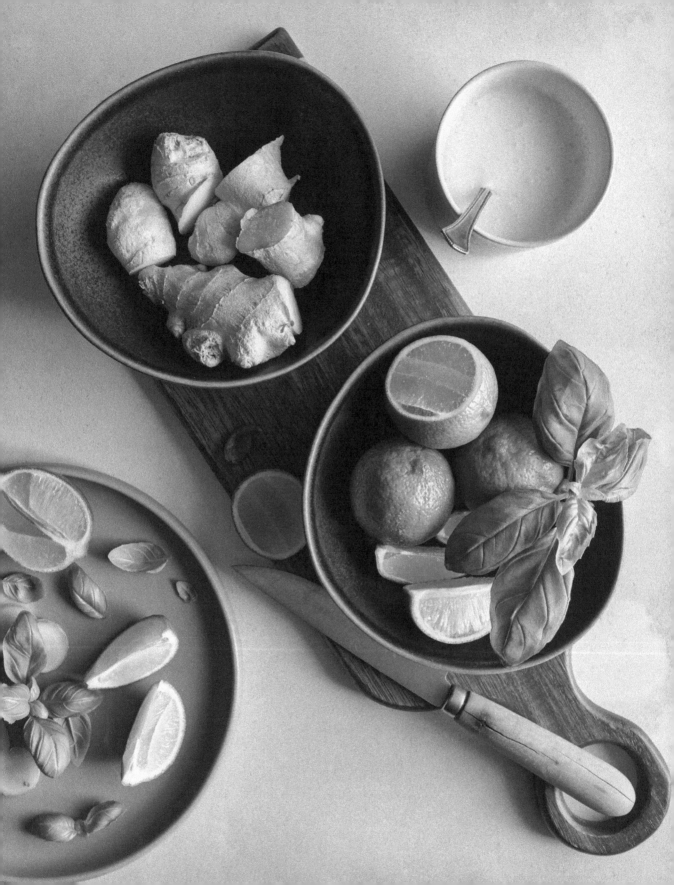

COCONUT MILK GINGER MARINATED PORK TENDERLOIN

SUPER QUICK

PREP TIME: 5 MINUTES | COOK TIME: 25 MINUTES
SERVES: 4

Coconut milk is a great add to a marinade because it's got a lot of fat, which can help add moisture to the meat. And adding in acidic lime juice creates the perfect tenderizing marinade. It's so delicious that you'll also want to use this marinade for your chicken or fish.

¼ cup coconut oil, divided

1½ pounds boneless pork chops, about ¾ inch thick

1 tablespoon grated fresh ginger

2 teaspoons minced garlic

1 cup coconut milk

1 teaspoon chopped fresh basil

Juice of 1 lime

½ cup shredded unsweetened coconut

1. **Brown the pork.** In a large skillet over medium heat, warm 2 tablespoons of the coconut oil. Add the pork chops to the skillet and brown them all over, turning them several times, about 10 minutes in total.

2. **Braise the pork.** Move the pork to the side of the skillet and add the remaining 2 tablespoons of coconut oil. Add the ginger and garlic and sauté until they've softened, about 2 minutes. Stir in the coconut milk, basil, and lime juice and move the pork back to the center of the skillet. Cover the skillet and simmer until the pork is just cooked through and very tender, 12 to 15 minutes.

3. **Serve.** Divide the pork chops between four plates and top them with the shredded coconut.

Tip: Stay away from light coconut milk because it will throw off the perfect macros in this recipe and will not make the same luscious sauce that's created by full-fat coconut milk.

PER SERVING
Macronutrients: Fat: 70%; Protein: 25%; Carbs: 5%
Calories: 479; Total fat: 38g; Total carbs: 6g; Fiber: 3g;
Net carbs: 3g; Sodium: 318mg; Protein: 32g

GRILLED PORK CHOPS WITH GREEK SALSA

SUPER QUICK | FULL GUIDO
PREP TIME: 15 MINUTES, PLUS MARINATING TIME | COOK TIME: 15 MINUTES
SERVES: 4

Salsa always makes a dish eye-popping and fresh-looking, thanks to all the bright colors and different textures. You can probably picture yourself eating these chops sitting on an outdoor patio. I mean, that's what I always picture when I'm making them. Anyway, definitely try this salsa with fish, chicken, and beef, too.

¼ cup good-quality olive oil, divided

1 tablespoon red wine vinegar

3 teaspoons chopped fresh oregano, divided

1 teaspoon minced garlic

4 (4-ounce) bone-less center-cut loin pork chops

½ cup halved cherry tomatoes

½ yellow bell pepper, diced

½ English cucumber, chopped

¼ red onion, chopped

1 tablespoon balsamic vinegar

Sea salt, for seasoning

Freshly ground black pepper, for seasoning

1. **Marinate the pork.** In a medium bowl, stir together 3 tablespoons of the olive oil, the vinegar, 2 teaspoons of the oregano, and the garlic. Add the pork chops to the bowl, turning them to get them coated with the marinade. Cover the bowl and place it in the refrigerator for 30 minutes.

2. **Make the salsa.** While the pork is marinating, in a medium bowl, stir together the remaining 1 tablespoon of olive oil, the tomatoes, yellow bell pepper, cucumber, red onion, vinegar, and the remaining 1 teaspoon of oregano. Season the salsa with salt and pepper. Set the bowl aside.

3. **Grill the pork chops.** Heat a grill to medium-high heat. Remove the pork chops from the marinade and grill them until just cooked through, 6 to 8 minutes per side.

4. **Serve.** Rest the pork for 5 minutes. Divide the pork between four plates and serve them with a generous scoop of the salsa.

Tip: The salsa can be made 2 days ahead and stored in the refrigerator in a sealed container until you are ready to serve this attractive dish. Let it come to room temperature before spooning it on the grilled pork.

PER SERVING
Macronutrients: Fat: 60%; Protein: 34%; Carbs: 6%
Calories: 277; Total fat: 19g; Total carbs: 4g; Fiber: 1g;
Net carbs: 3g; Sodium: 257mg; Protein: 25g

GRILLED HERBED PORK KEBABS

SUPER QUICK | FULL GUIDO

PREP TIME: 10 MINUTES, PLUS MARINATING TIME | COOK TIME: 15 MINUTES

SERVES: 4

Kebabs are a lot of fun. They're fun to eat, they look festive on a plate, and they're really easy to make. If you use wooden skewers, soak them in water for at least half an hour beforehand so they don't catch fire when you place them on the grill. They still might smolder a little, but they won't burn through. Metal skewers are the best, just be careful removing them because the metal will heat right down to the handle.

¼ cup good-quality olive oil

1 tablespoon minced garlic

2 teaspoons dried oregano

1 teaspoon dried basil

1 teaspoon dried parsley

½ teaspoon sea salt

¼ teaspoon freshly ground black pepper

1 (1-pound) pork tenderloin, cut into 1½-inch pieces

1. **Marinate the pork.** In a medium bowl, stir together the olive oil, garlic, oregano, basil, parsley, salt, and pepper. Add the pork pieces and toss to coat them in the marinade. Cover the bowl and place it in the refrigerator for 2 to 4 hours.

2. **Make the kebabs.** Divide the pork pieces between four skewers, making sure to not crowd the meat.

3. **Grill the kebabs.** Preheat your grill to medium-high heat. Grill the skewers for about 12 minutes, turning to cook all sides of the pork, until the pork is cooked through.

4. **Serve.** Rest the skewers for 5 minutes. Divide the skewers between four plates and serve them immediately.

Tip: Add whole button mushrooms, zucchini chunks, red onion, and bell pepper pieces for a full meal on a skewer. Keep a little space between the vegetables and meat on the skewers so that everything cooks evenly and thoroughly. This addition of low-carb vegetables will add 3 to 5 grams of carbs per serving.

PER SERVING
Macronutrients: Fat: 60%; Protein: 39%; Carbs: 1%
Calories: 261; Total fat: 18g; Total carbs: 1g; Fiber: 0g;
Net carbs: 1g; Sodium: 60mg; Protein: 24g

ITALIAN SAUSAGE BROCCOLI SAUTÉ

SUPER QUICK | FULL GUIDO

PREP TIME: 10 MINUTES | COOK TIME: 20 MINUTES

SERVES: 4

My grandfather used to make his own sausage. I remember all the meat sitting out on the table and the machine he had that would grind up that meat and turn it into sausages. I like to think of him when I make this dish, even though I'm using the sausage in a different way. The truth is, I like how easy this is to make. It has very few ingredients, but it still packs a punch of flavor. Broccoli is a good combo with sausage, and it's got an earthy flavor when it's lightly caramelized.

2 tablespoons
good-quality olive oil

1 pound Italian sausage
meat, hot or mild

4 cups small
broccoli florets

1 tablespoon
minced garlic

Freshly ground black
pepper, for seasoning

1. **Cook the sausage.** In a large skillet over medium heat, warm the olive oil. Add the sausage and sauté it until it's cooked through, 8 to 10 minutes. Transfer the sausage to a plate with a slotted spoon and set the plate aside.

2. **Sauté the vegetables.** Add the broccoli to the skillet and sauté it until it's tender, about 6 minutes. Stir in the garlic and sauté for another 3 minutes.

3. **Finish the dish.** Return the sausage to the skillet and toss to combine it with the other ingredients. Season the mixture with pepper.

4. **Serve.** Divide the mixture between four plates and serve it immediately.

Swap: This can be made with cooked sausage cut into ½-inch pieces instead of meat out of the casings. Just sauté the cooked pieces and prepare the recipe the same way.

PER SERVING

Macronutrients: Fat: 79%; Protein: 16%; Carbs: 5%
Calories: 486; Total fat: 43g; Total carbs: 7g; Fiber: 2g;
Net carbs: 5g; Sodium: 513mg; Protein: 19g

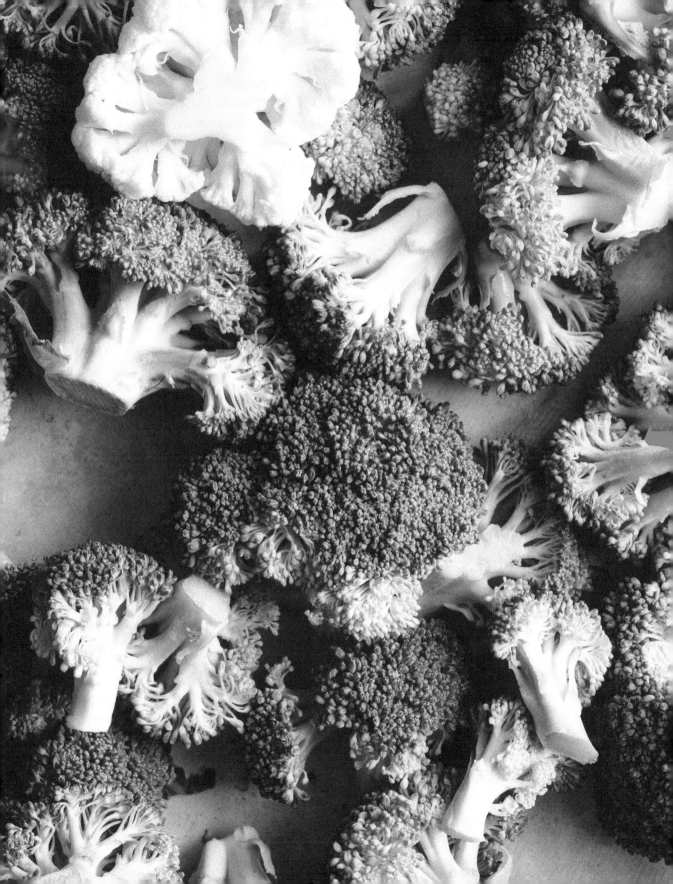

CLASSIC SAUSAGE AND PEPPERS

FULL GUIDO

PREP TIME: 10 MINUTES | COOK TIME: 35 MINUTES

SERVES: 6

Sausage and pepper heroes are a big staple of the Jersey Shore boardwalk. But that's actually not the reason I love the combo. I grew up eating sausage and peppers served on a hero, which always felt like the perfect comfort food. Obviously I had to make a keto version without the processed carbs, and after some trial and error, I realized the sausage and peppers didn't even need bread or pasta—they're great on their own. Also, in my opinion, sausage is a brilliant way to use up all of an animal, which is a responsible way to eat because you're not wasting anything.

1½ pounds sweet Italian sausages (or hot if you prefer)

2 tablespoons good-quality olive oil

1 red bell pepper, cut into thin strips

1 yellow bell pepper, cut into thin strips

1 orange bell pepper, cut into thin strips

1 red onion, thinly sliced

1 tablespoon minced garlic

½ cup white wine

Sea salt, for seasoning

Freshly ground black pepper, for seasoning

1. **Cook the sausage.** Preheat a grill to medium-high and grill the sausages, turning them several times, until they're cooked through, about 12 minutes in total. Let the sausages rest for 15 minutes and then cut them into 2-inch pieces.

2. **Sauté the vegetables.** In a large skillet over medium-high heat, warm the olive oil. Add the red, yellow, and orange bell peppers, and the red onion and garlic and sauté until they're tender, about 10 minutes.

3. **Finish the dish.** Add the sausage to the skillet along with the white wine and sauté for 10 minutes.

4. **Serve.** Divide the mixture between four plates, season it with salt and pepper, and serve.

Tip: Don't skip resting the sausages or you could risk getting burned by spurting juices. There will be some juice when you cut the sausages, but most will stay in the meat where it belongs.

Swap: If you want to vary it up, throw in a couple cups of chopped tomatoes with the white wine.

PER SERVING
Macronutrients: Fat: 80%; Protein: 16%; Carbs: 4%
Calories: 450; Total fat: 40g; Total carbs: 5g; Fiber: 1g;
Net carbs: 4g; Sodium: 554mg; Protein: 17g

LEMON-INFUSED PORK RIB ROAST

FULL GUIDO

PREP TIME: 10 MINUTES, PLUS MARINATING TIME | COOK TIME: 1 HOUR
SERVES: 6

Pork rib roast, or rack of pork, is from the rib area of the loin. It's got slightly more fat than other cuts in that area, so it's more flavorful, and great for keto. Don't worry about the whole garlic cloves you're inserting in the meat being too much—they will roast slowly, becoming buttery and tender with a mellow taste. If you love garlic like I do, you can insert even more cloves.

¼ cup good-quality olive oil

Zest and juice of 1 lemon

Zest and juice of 1 orange

4 rosemary sprigs, lightly crushed

4 thyme sprigs, lightly crushed

1 (4-bone) pork rib roast, about 2½ pounds

6 garlic cloves, peeled

Sea salt, for seasoning

Freshly ground black pepper, for seasoning

1. **Make the marinade.** In a large bowl, combine the olive oil, lemon zest, lemon juice, orange zest, orange juice, rosemary sprigs, and thyme sprigs.

2. **Marinate the roast.** Use a small knife to make six 1-inch-deep slits in the fatty side of the roast. Stuff the garlic cloves in the slits. Put the roast in the bowl with the marinade and turn it to coat it well with the marinade. Cover the bowl and refrigerate it overnight, turning the roast in the marinade several times.

3. **Preheat the oven.** Set the oven temperature to 350°F.

4. **Roast the pork.** Remove the pork from the marinade and season it with salt and pepper, then put it in a baking dish and let it come to room temperature. Roast the pork until it's cooked through (145°F to 160°F internal temperature), about 1 hour. Throw out any leftover marinade.

5. **Serve.** Let the pork rest for 10 minutes, then cut it into slices and arrange the slices on a platter. Serve it warm.

Tip: You can easily double this recipe for a spectacular holiday meat for extended family. Cook the roast for 2 hours, or about 25 minutes per pound.

PER SERVING
Macronutrients: Fat: 70%; Protein: 29%; Carbs: 1%
Calories: 403; Total fat: 30g; Total carbs: 1g; Fiber: 0g;
Net carbs: 1g; Sodium: 113mg; Protein: 30g

PORK MEATBALL PARMESAN

FULL GUIDO

PREP TIME: 15 MINUTES | COOK TIME: 30 MINUTES

SERVES: 6

"Parmesan" here just means this dish uses the tomato sauce and melted cheese you usually find on top of chicken Parmesan. This meatball dish works well as a snack or a meal. And if you want a bigger meal, it can be served with zucchini or vegetable noodles. Sometimes when I make this, I like to pair it with a side of ricotta cheese to go full-on Italian.

FOR THE MEATBALLS

1¼ pounds ground pork

½ cup almond flour

½ cup Parmesan cheese

1 egg, lightly beaten

1 tablespoon chopped fresh parsley

1 teaspoon minced garlic

1 teaspoon chopped fresh oregano

¼ teaspoon sea salt

⅛ teaspoon freshly ground black pepper

2 tablespoons good-quality olive oil

FOR THE PARMIGIANA

1 cup sugar-free tomato sauce

1 cup shredded mozzarella cheese

TO MAKE THE MEATBALLS

1. **Make the meatballs.** In a large bowl, mix together the ground pork, almond flour, Parmesan, egg, parsley, garlic, oregano, salt, and pepper until everything is well mixed. Roll the pork mixture into 1½-inch meatballs.

2. **Cook the meatballs.** In a large skillet over medium-high heat, warm the olive oil. Add the meatballs to the skillet and cook them, turning them several times, until they're completely cooked through, about 15 minutes in total.

TO MAKE THE PARMIGIANA

1. **Preheat the oven.** Set the oven temperature to 350°F.

2. **Assemble the parmigiana.** Transfer the meatballs to a 9-by-9-inch baking dish and top them with the tomato sauce. Sprinkle with the mozzarella and bake for 15 minutes or until the cheese is melted and golden.

3. **Serve.** Divide the meatballs and sauce between six bowls and serve it immediately.

Tip: If you want to make this ahead of time, you can. When you're done, instead of serving it, just put it in an oven-safe container, cover it, and freeze it for up to one month. Then thaw it in the fridge overnight and pop it in the oven for an easy meal.

Swap: Bison, venison, beef, or lamb would all be delicious instead of pork for these juicy meatballs. You can also mix different combinations to create the perfect palate-pleasing taste.

PER SERVING
Macronutrients: Fat: 73%; Protein: 26%; Carbs: 1%
Calories: 403; Total fat: 32g; Total carbs: 1g; Fiber: 0g;
Net carbs: 1g; Sodium: 351mg; Protein: 25g

T-BONE STEAK WITH CITRUS MARINADE

SUPER QUICK | FULL GUIDO
PREP TIME: 5 MINUTES, PLUS MARINATING TIME | COOK TIME: 15 MINUTES
SERVES: 4

T-bone steaks are a great combo of two prime cuts of meat: a strip of the top loin and a chunk of tenderloin. One of the best methods for cooking a T-bone is grilling, because all the fat marbling keeps the meat moist, and the bone is an easy area to flip the steak without accidentally piercing the meat. Make sure you position the filet part of the steak farthest away from the hottest part of the grill, because it cooks the fastest.

¼ cup good-quality olive oil

¼ cup freshly squeezed lime juice

2 tablespoons balsamic vinegar

2 tablespoons freshly squeezed orange juice

1 tablespoon minced garlic

1 tablespoon finely chopped fresh basil

4 T-bone steaks (about 1½ pounds total)

1. **Marinate the beef.** In a medium bowl, stir together the olive oil, lime juice, vinegar, orange juice, garlic, and basil. Pour the marinade into a resealable plastic bag and add the steaks to the bag. Squeeze out the excess air and seal the bag. Refrigerate the steak to marinate for 30 minutes.

2. **Grill the steak.** Preheat the grill to medium-high heat. Remove the steak from the marinade and grill it for 6 to 7 minutes per side for medium (140°F internal temperature) or until it's done the way you like it. Throw out any leftover marinade.

3. **Rest and serve.** Let the steak rest for 10 minutes. Divide the steaks between four plates and serve them immediately.

Tip: If you want rare steaks, let the meat get to room temperature before grilling so that there are no colder spots in the center of the steaks, and they will stay juicy.

PER SERVING
Macronutrients: Fat: 72%; Protein: 26%; Carbs: 2%
Calories: 524; Total fat: 42g; Total carbs: 3g; Fiber: 0g;
Net carbs: 3g; Sodium: 91mg; Protein: 32g

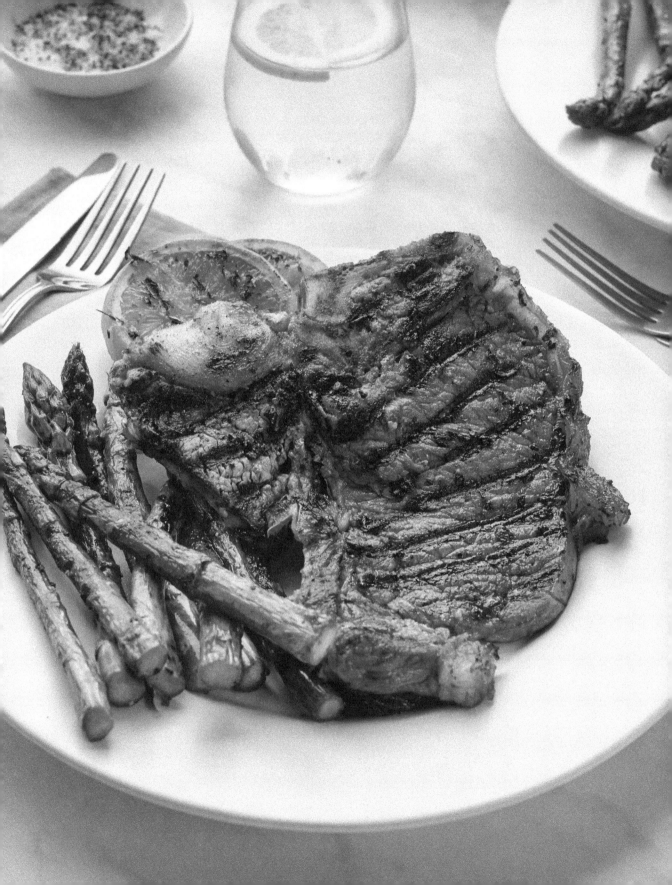

SPICY FRIED BEEF WITH CHILES

FULL GUIDO

PREP TIME: 10 MINUTES, PLUS MARINATING TIME | COOK TIME: 1 HOUR, 45 MINUTES

SERVES: 4

The habanero chile takes this flavor-packed dish to the spicy side of dinner, but you can serve it with a plate of sliced cucumbers, which will help cut the heat. You can also use chiles that are less spicy, like jalapeños or dried guajillo chiles, if you prefer.

1½ tablespoons minced garlic

1 tablespoon grated fresh ginger

1 shallot, finely chopped

1 teaspoon chili powder

1 teaspoon ground cinnamon

1 teaspoon ground cumin

½ teaspoon ground coriander

Pinch cayenne pepper

1½ pounds beef chuck, cut into 1-inch chunks

¼ cup good-quality olive oil

1 onion, peeled and thinly sliced

1 red bell pepper, thinly sliced

1 habanero pepper, minced

1 cup Beef Bone Broth (page 236)

1 cup shredded unsweetened coconut

½ cup sour cream

1. **Marinate the beef.** In a medium bowl, stir together the garlic, ginger, shallot, chili powder, cinnamon, cumin, coriander, and cayenne to form a paste. Add the beef to the bowl and massage the paste into the pieces of beef. Cover the bowl and marinate the beef in the refrigerator for at least 4 hours.

2. **Brown the beef.** In a large saucepan over medium-high heat, warm the olive oil. Add the beef to the pan and sauté it until it has browned, about 10 minutes in total.

3. **Sauté the vegetables.** Add the onion, red bell pepper, and habanero pepper to the pan and sauté until they're tender, about 4 minutes.

4. **Braise the beef.** Add the beef broth and bring the liquid to a boil, then reduce the heat to low and simmer until the beef is very tender and the liquid reduces, about 1½ hours. Add more broth if the beef is not tender enough.

5. **Finish and serve.** Stir in the coconut and serve the beef topped with the sour cream.

Tip: To make this dish more weeknight friendly, mix together the marinade and meat in a resealable plastic bag and put it in the freezer. The night before you want to make the dish, place the bag in the refrigerator. By the time you get home from work the next day, the meat will be ready to cook.

PER SERVING
Macronutrients: Fat: 62%; Protein: 31%; Carbs: 7%
Calories: 528; Total fat: 37g; Total carbs: 8g; Fiber: 4g;
Net carbs: 4g; Sodium: 275mg; Protein: 41g

FLAKY BEEF EMPANADAS

FULL GUIDO

PREP TIME: 30 MINUTES | COOK TIME: 25 MINUTES

SERVES: 6

Empanadas originally come from Spain and Portugal, and the name comes from the word *empanar*, which means "to wrap in bread." But guess what? You don't need the bread. My recipe will give you a delicious dough that's better. After eating these, you won't want regular ones, I promise. You can fill these handheld pies with so many options, like lamb, chicken, sausage, cheese, ham, or beef like I do in this recipe. I eat these all the time—as a meal at home, a convenient snack when I'm on set shooting *Jersey Shore*, or even as a quick, on-the-go breakfast when I've got a busy day ahead and have to run out the door.

FOR THE DOUGH

1 cup mozzarella cheese, shredded

5 tablespoons cream cheese

¾ cup almond flour

2 tablespoons coconut milk

1 tablespoon coconut flour

1 egg, lightly beaten

1 teaspoon garlic powder

½ teaspoon sea salt

TO MAKE THE DOUGH

1. **Melt the cheeses.** In a small saucepan over low heat, melt the mozzarella and cream cheese together, stirring often. Remove the pan from the heat.

2. **Mix the dough.** Transfer the cheese mixture to a medium bowl and stir in the almond flour, coconut milk, coconut flour, egg, garlic powder, and salt until everything is well blended and the mixture holds together in a ball. Cover the bowl with plastic wrap, pressing it down onto the surface of the dough, and place the bowl in the refrigerator for 30 minutes.

FOR THE FILLING

¼ cup grass-fed butter

1 pound grass-fed
    ground beef

1 onion, chopped

1 tablespoon
    minced garlic

2 tablespoons sugar-free
    tomato paste

2 teaspoons
    ground cumin

2 teaspoons
    dried oregano

1 teaspoon chili powder

Sea salt, for seasoning

Freshly ground black
    pepper, for seasoning

TO MAKE THE FILLING

1. **Cook the beef.** In a large skillet over medium-high heat, melt the butter. Add the beef and cook it until it's browned, about 7 minutes.

2. **Finish the filling.** Add the onion and garlic and sauté until they've softened, about 4 minutes. Stir in the tomato paste, cumin, oregano, and chili powder. Season the filling with salt and pepper and set it aside to cool.

TO MAKE THE EMPANADAS

1. **Preheat the oven.** Set the oven temperature to 425°F. Line a baking sheet with parchment paper.

2. **Cut the dough.** Spread some parchment paper on your work surface. Press the dough out into a thin layer on the paper, then cut the dough into 12 (3-inch) circles.

3. **Fill the dough.** Spoon the filling equally onto the middle of each dough circle. Fold the dough over and press the edges together using a fork to seal them.

CONTINUED ▶

4. **Bake.** Transfer the empanadas to the baking sheet and bake them for 10 to 12 minutes until they're golden brown.

5. **Serve.** Divide the empanadas between six plates and serve them immediately.

Tip: Double up the recipe and freeze them. This will make your life so easy. Place the unbaked filled empanadas on a baking sheet and freeze them for an hour. Transfer the frozen empanadas to a resealable plastic container and freeze for up to one month. Thaw as many of the empanadas as you like in the refrigerator and bake by following the recipe.

PER SERVING
Macronutrients: Fat: 76%; Protein: 20%; Carbs: 4%
Calories: 436; Total fat: 38g; Total carbs: 4g; Fiber: 1g;
Net carbs: 3g; Sodium: 229mg; Protein: 19g

BISTECCA ALLA FIORENTINA

SUPER QUICK | FULL GUIDO

PREP TIME: 10 MINUTES | COOK TIME: 15 MINUTES

SERVES: 4

Porterhouse steaks are basically oversize T-bones and are meant to serve two people—or one very hungry person. To hit the porterhouse designation, the cut has to have a tenderloin section that's 1¼ inches at its widest point. Look for a good marbling of white fat, especially in the loin section, and avoid cuts with yellow fat.

2 (1-inch-thick) bone-in porterhouse steaks, about 2 pounds

6 tablespoons good-quality olive oil, divided

Sea salt, for seasoning

Freshly ground black pepper, for seasoning

½ cup white wine

2 rosemary sprigs

Lemon wedges, for serving

1. **Preheat the grill.** Preheat the grill to high heat.

2. **Prepare the steaks.** Rub the steaks with 2 tablespoons of the olive oil and season them generously with salt and pepper.

3. **Prepare the basting liquid.** In a small bowl, stir together the white wine and the remaining 4 tablespoons of olive oil.

4. **Grill the steaks.** Using the rosemary sprigs as basters, baste the steaks on both sides with the wine mixture. Grill the steaks, flipping them once, until they're seared on both sides, 6 to 8 minutes in total (125°F internal temperature) for medium rare.

5. **Serve.** Let the steaks rest for 10 minutes, then divide them between four plates, and serve them with lemon wedges.

Tip: Make sure your rosemary sprigs are fresh and have lots of needles on the end to create the perfect flexible marinade mop. Older rosemary sprigs will be stiffer and will impart less flavor to the steaks.

PER SERVING
Macronutrients: Fat: 71%; Protein: 26%; Carbs: 3%
Calories: 569; Total fat: 45g; Total carbs: 0g; Fiber: 0g;
Net carbs: 0g; Sodium: 238mg; Protein: 35g

SIMPLE LIVER AND ONIONS

FULL GUIDO

PREP TIME: 10 MINUTES | COOK TIME: 25 MINUTES

SERVES: 4

Not everyone likes the idea of eating liver, I know. But this is a classic combo that you can find at so many places, from roadside diners to Michelin star restaurants. The dish even has its own holiday—May 10 is National Liver and Onions Day—so if you need an excuse to make this recipe, May 10 is your day. Some people might be grossed out by this combo, but I really love it. Test it out, you may be surprised. Liver is a superfood, so in addition to tasting good, it's really healthy. If you're still not convinced, try adding chopped bacon to the onions and cook it until it's crispy for extra flavor and texture.

½ cup grass-fed butter

¼ cup extra-virgin olive oil

2 onions, thinly sliced

½ cup white wine

1 pound calf's liver, trimmed and cut into strips

1 tablespoon balsamic vinegar

2 tablespoons chopped fresh parsley

Sea salt, for seasoning

Freshly ground black pepper, for seasoning

1. **Sauté the onions.** In a large skillet over medium heat, warm the butter and olive oil. Add the onions to the skillet and sauté them until they've softened, about 5 minutes. Stir in the white wine and reduce the heat to medium-low. Cover the skillet and cook, stirring frequently, until the onions are very soft and lightly browned, about 15 minutes. Transfer the onions with a slotted spoon to a plate.

2. **Cook the liver.** Increase the heat to high and stir in the liver strips and the vinegar. Sauté the liver until it's done the way you like it, about 4 minutes for medium rare.

3. **Finish the dish.** Return the onions to the skillet along with the parsley, stirring to combine them. Season the liver and onions with salt and pepper.

4. **Serve.** Divide the liver and onions between four
    plates and serve immediately.

Tip: If you like the nutritional aspect of liver but you
find the taste is a little strong, try soaking the liver
in lemon juice or kefir to cut down on the metallic
or "iron" taste.

PER SERVING
Macronutrients: Fat: 72%; Protein: 20%; Carbs: 8%
Calories: 497; Total fat: 40g; Total carbs: 8g; Fiber: 3g;
Net carbs: 5g; Sodium: 103mg; Protein: 23g

GRILLED SKIRT STEAK WITH JALAPEÑO COMPOUND BUTTER

SUPER QUICK | FULL GUIDO

PREP TIME: 10 MINUTES, PLUS CHILLING TIME | COOK TIME: 10 MINUTES

SERVES: 4

Fun fact: In most of the US, skirt steak used to be looked at as "bad meat" that should be disregarded. Now it's on the menu at many of the fanciest steak houses. Go figure. This is hands-down my favorite steak to make at home. Skirt steak is a very flavorful cut of beef, but it can be tough. That's why grilling is a good option—and I love to grill. The thing about skirt steak that makes it so tasty is that it has a good amount of fat on it, so it stays juicy. Just make sure to use a very hot grill when you cook it, and slice it very thinly across the grain, so it's tender.

¼ cup unsalted grass-fed butter, at room temperature

½ jalapeño pepper, seeded and minced very finely

Zest and juice of ½ lime

½ teaspoon sea salt

4 (4-ounce) skirt steaks

1 tablespoon olive oil

Sea salt, for seasoning

Freshly ground black pepper, for seasoning

1. **Make the compound butter.** In a medium bowl, stir together the butter, jalapeño pepper, lime zest, lime juice, and salt until everything is well combined. Lay a piece of plastic wrap on a clean work surface and spoon the butter mixture into the middle. Form the butter into a log about 1 inch thick by folding the plastic wrap over the butter and twisting the two ends in opposite directions. Roll the butter log on the counter to smooth the edges and put it in the freezer until it's very firm, about 4 hours.

2. **Grill the steak.** Preheat the grill to high heat. Lightly oil the steaks with the olive oil and season them lightly with salt and pepper. Grill the steaks for about 5 minutes per side for medium (140°F internal temperature) or until they're done the way you like them.

3. Rest and serve. Let the steaks rest for 10 minutes and serve them sliced across the grain, topped with a thick slice of the compound butter.

Tip: Compound butters can be made weeks in advance and stored in the freezer. Just cut off a generous chunk for steaks, pork, chicken, or vegetables whenever you need it. You can also put the butter in ice cube trays and freeze it. Transfer the frozen butter cubes to a sealed plastic bag and store in the freezer for up to three months.

PER SERVING
Macronutrients: Fat: 71%; Protein: 29%; Carbs: 0%
Calories: 404 Total fat: 32g; Total carbs: 0g; Fiber: 0g;
Net carbs: 0g; Sodium: 292mg; Protein: 29g

RIB-EYE WITH CHIMICHURRI SAUCE

SUPER QUICK

PREP TIME: 15 MINUTES, PLUS RESTING TIME | COOK TIME: 15 MINUTES

SERVES: 4

Rib-eye steaks are probably my favorite thing to order at a restaurant, so I decided I should learn how to make them at home. Rib-eyes (also called Delmonico steaks) come from the cut of beef that's a prime rib when it's left whole. Rib-eyes can have the bone on or off, and my recipe is bone off. (Although I do love a good bone to gnaw on!) There's really generous fat marbling in rib-eyes, especially around the center muscle, so they're perfect for grilling. If you do decide to use bone-on steaks, remember that the area closest to the bone cooks slower, so it'll still be medium rare while the rest of the steak is medium.

FOR THE CHIMICHURRI

½ cup good-quality olive oil

½ cup finely chopped fresh parsley

2 tablespoons red wine vinegar

2 tablespoons finely chopped fresh cilantro

1½ tablespoons minced garlic

1 tablespoon finely chopped chile pepper

½ teaspoon sea salt

¼ teaspoon freshly ground black pepper

FOR THE STEAK

4 (5-ounce) rib-eye steaks

1 tablespoon good-quality olive oil

Sea salt, for seasoning

Freshly ground black pepper, for seasoning

TO MAKE THE CHIMICHURRI

Make the chimichurri. In a medium bowl, stir together the olive oil, parsley, vinegar, cilantro, garlic, chile, salt, and pepper. Let it stand for 15 minutes to mellow the flavors.

TO MAKE THE STEAK

1. **Prepare the steaks.** Let the steaks come to room temperature and lightly oil them with the olive oil and season them with salt and pepper.

2. **Grill the steaks.** Preheat the grill to high heat. Grill the steaks for 6 to 7 minutes per side for medium (140°F internal temperature) or until they're done the way you like them.

3. Rest and serve. Let the steaks rest for 10 minutes and then serve them topped with generous spoonfuls of the chimichurri sauce.

Tip: Chimichurri sauce is not just delicious with steak; it can be spooned over vegetables, eggs, chicken, fish, and pork. You can even stir it into sour cream for a flavorful dip.

PER SERVING
Macronutrients: Fat: 75%; Protein: 24%; Carbs: 1%
Calories: 503; Total fat: 42g; Total Carbs: 1g; Fiber: 0g;
Net carbs: 1g; Sodium: 385mg; Protein: 29g

BEEF SAUSAGE MEAT LOAF

FULL GUIDO

PREP TIME: 10 MINUTES | COOK TIME: 1 HOUR, 15 MINUTES

SERVES: 6

Meat loaf is one of the easiest, tastiest meals to prepare. And a finished meat loaf is so versatile—warm or cold, it's still delicious. If you're not serving this to your family or friends and it's just for you, cook the meat loaf in a muffin pan instead of a loaf pan. Then you can pop out perfectly formed "muffins" of individual servings and store them in bags in the fridge or freezer for the future. Cooking it that way also means you'll get delicious browning all the way around each portion, and the "muffins" hold together better than slices.

1½ pounds Italian sausage meat

1 pound grass-fed ground beef

½ cup almond flour

¼ cup heavy (whipping) cream

1 egg, lightly beaten

½ onion, finely chopped

½ red bell pepper, chopped

2 teaspoons minced garlic

1 teaspoon dried oregano

¼ teaspoon sea salt

⅛ teaspoon freshly ground black pepper

1. **Preheat the oven.** Set the oven temperature to 400°F.

2. **Make the meat loaf.** In a large bowl, mix together the sausage, ground beef, almond flour, cream, egg, onion, red bell pepper, garlic, oregano, salt, and pepper until everything is well combined. Press the mixture into a 9-inch loaf pan.

3. **Bake.** Bake for 1 hour to 1 hour and 15 minutes, or until the meat loaf is cooked through. Drain off and throw out any grease and let the meat loaf stand for 10 minutes.

4. **Serve.** Cut the meat loaf into six slices, divide them between six plates, and serve it immediately.

Tip: If your ground beef has a higher fat percentage, tip out some grease halfway through cooking and once again before it finishes cooking.

PER SERVING
Macronutrients: Fat: 78%; Protein: 21%; Carbs: 1%
Calories: 394; Total fat: 34g; Total carbs: 1g; Fiber: 0g;
Net carbs: 1g; Sodium: 325mg; Protein: 19g

JUICY NO-FAIL BURGER

SUPER QUICK

PREP TIME: 10 MINUTES | COOK TIME: 15 MINUTES

SERVES: 4

Burgers are a staple keto dish at every meal, even breakfast—and with a whole bunch of different toppings. My trick to a great burger is using high-quality ground beef with the perfect amount of fat. Grass-fed beef is slightly leaner than factory-raised in some cases, so if your beef is really lean, add some chopped bacon to up the fat content. These burgers can be put together and laid on a baking tray and frozen individually, then packed in a container so you can cook them right from frozen.

1 pound grass-fed ground beef

1 egg, lightly beaten

½ onion, finely chopped

1 teaspoon minced garlic

1 teaspoon Worcestershire sauce

1 teaspoon dried parsley

¼ teaspoon sea salt

⅛ teaspoon freshly ground black pepper

1 tablespoon olive oil

1. **Make the burgers.** In a medium bowl, combine the ground beef, egg, onion, garlic, Worcestershire sauce, parsley, salt, and pepper until everything is well mixed. Form the mixture into four equal patties, each about ¾ inch thick. Lightly oil the patties with olive oil.

2. **Grill the burgers.** Preheat the grill to medium heat. Grill the burgers, turning them once, until they're just cooked through (160°F internal temperature), about 8 minutes per side.

3. **Serve.** Let the burgers rest for 5 minutes, then serve them immediately.

Tip: Whenever possible, use fresh ground beef from a butcher rather than prepackaged meat because vacuum packing can suck moisture out of the meat, which makes for a drier burger.

PER SERVING
Macronutrients: Fat: 77%; Protein: 22%; Carbs: 1%
Calories: 379; Total fat: 33g; Total carbs: 1g; Fiber: 0g;
Net carbs: 1g; Sodium: 238mg; Protein: 19g

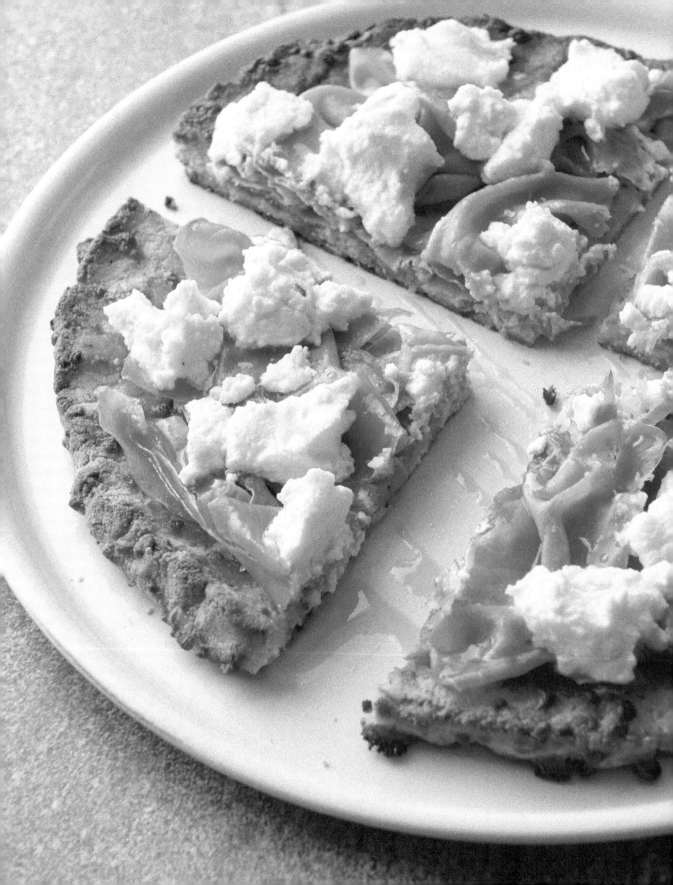

PIZZA WITH PROSCIUTTO, RICOTTA, AND TRUFFLE OIL

SUPER QUICK | FULL GUIDO
PREP TIME: 15 MINUTES | COOK TIME: 7 MINUTES
SERVES: 4

Many people have seen the video clip of me from *Jersey Shore*, where I'm peeling the cheese off my pizza and eating that cheese plain. No one can say I'm not committed to eating keto! Luckily, with this recipe, I can eat the whole pizza because of the special keto dough. This recipe is one of my favorites, and after my mom and I made this on *Good Morning America*, people got so excited that I knew I had to include it in this book. This pizza is really good and makes me feel kinda fancy when I eat it, since truffle oil is a lot more sophisticated than heaps of melted cheese.

FOR THE PIZZA CRUST

1¾ cups shredded mozzarella cheese

3 tablespoons plain cream cheese

1 cup almond flour

½ teaspoon dried basil

½ teaspoon dried oregano

Pinch sea salt

1 egg, lightly beaten

Olive oil cooking spray

ingredients continue on next page

TO MAKE THE PIZZA CRUST

1. **Preheat the oven.** Set the oven temperature to broil.

2. **Melt the cheeses.** Stir together the mozzarella and cream cheese in a large microwave-safe bowl and microwave on high for 1 minute. Stir the cheeses and heat them again for 30 seconds to 1 minute until they're completely melted.

3. **Add the dry ingredients.** Stir in the almond flour, basil, oregano, and salt until everything is well mixed and set it aside to cool to room temperature, about 10 minutes.

4. **Finish the dough.** When the mixture has cooled enough that it won't cook the egg, mix in the egg until it's well blended, then gather the dough into a ball.

CONTINUED

FOR THE PIZZA

6 ounces prosciutto

8 ounces ricotta cheese

Truffle oil

5. **Roll the dough.** Lay a piece of parchment paper on a baking sheet and spray it lightly with olive oil. Place the dough on the sheet in the center and press it down with your fingers to form a disc until it is about ⅓ inch thick. It's fine if the dough looks rustic and not perfectly round.

6. **Broil the dough.** Broil the dough until it is golden and firm, about 4 minutes.

TO MAKE THE PIZZA

1. **Preheat the oven.** Preheat the oven to 425°F.

2. **Top the pizza.** Place the prosciutto over the pizza crust. Then use a small ice cream scoop to distribute about 6 scoops of ricotta cheese on top, evenly spacing the cheese mounds. Do not spread it out because the cheese will melt when baked. Drizzle the truffle oil with a spoon all over the pizza.

3. **Bake the pizza.** Place the pizza back in the oven and bake until the ricotta is melted, about 5 to 7 minutes.

4. **Serve.** Cut it into slices, and serve it immediately.

Tip: If you want to add flavor, you can add seasoning into your dough. I like to use Italian seasoning and spices.

Alternative method: You can also grill this pizza. Just follow this recipe, and after you top it, throw it on a medium-high heat grill, close the lid, and grill for 2-3 minutes.

Swap: Pizza toppings can be swapped out to create your favorite combinations in an unending variety. Mushrooms, chicken, shrimp, pesto, red pepper, onion, sundried tomato, and other types of cheese work beautifully. The nutrition info will change depending on what toppings you use in this dish.

PER SERVING
Macronutrients: Fat: 63%; Protein: 29%; Carbs: 8%
Calories: 446; Total fat: 31g; Total carbs: 10g; Fiber: 2g;
Net carbs: 8g; Sodium: 985mg; Protein: 32g

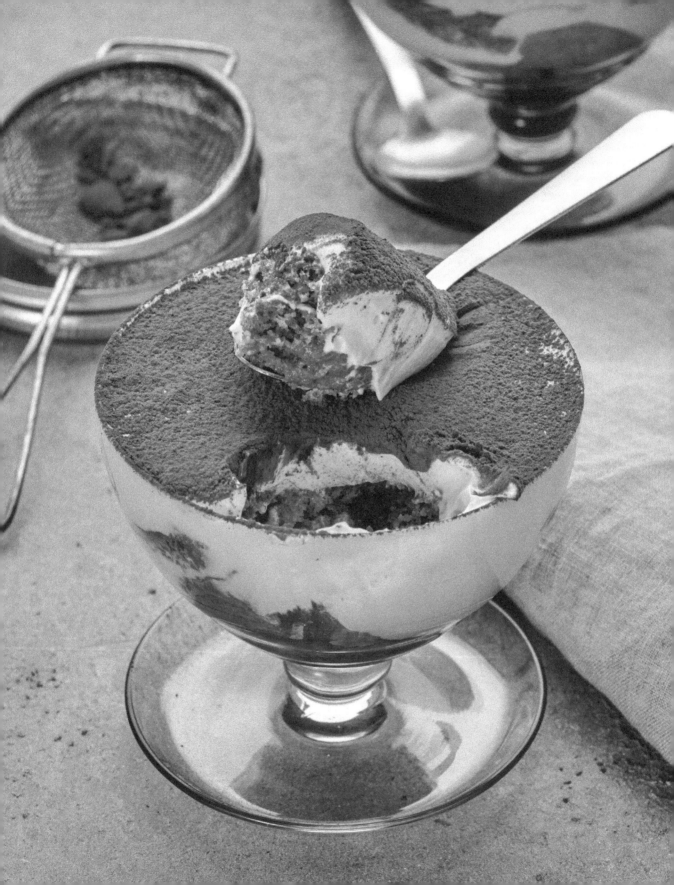

Desserts

One of the biggest excuses I hear for not doing keto is, "I'd miss desserts too much." Honestly, I get it. Desserts are the one food I miss the most while doing keto, too. Giving up that tiramisu after a big meal? That was hard for me. That's why I created these keto-friendly desserts, so you don't have to go without. That being said, these are still treats, rather than something to eat every day.

GOLDEN SESAME COOKIES

SUPER QUICK

PREP TIME: 10 MINUTES | COOK TIME: 15 MINUTES

MAKES 16 COOKIES

I like using golden sesame seeds for these delicious cookies instead of black ones, mostly because the golden ones come out looking the best. Even better, sesame seeds are really healthy since they can help lower cholesterol and cut the risk of high blood pressure.

1 cup almond flour

⅓ cup monk fruit sweetener, granulated form

¾ teaspoon baking powder

½ cup grass-fed butter, at room temperature

1 egg

1 teaspoon toasted sesame oil

½ cup sesame seeds

1. **Preheat the oven.** Set the oven temperature to 375°F. Line a baking sheet with parchment paper and set it aside.

2. **Mix the dry ingredients.** In a large bowl, mix together the almond flour, sweetener, and baking powder.

3. **Add the wet ingredients.** Add the butter, egg, and sesame oil to the dry ingredients and mix until everything is well blended.

4. **Form the cookies.** Roll the dough into 1½-inch balls and roll them in the sesame seeds. Place the cookies on the baking sheet about 2 inches apart and flatten them with your fingers so they are ½ inch thick.

5. **Bake the cookies.** Bake for 15 minutes, or until the cookies are golden brown. Transfer them to a wire rack and let them cool.

6. **Store.** Store the cookies in a sealed container in the refrigerator for up to five days, or in the freezer for up to one month.

Swap: Coconut oil can be used instead of butter for a rich nutty taste that complements the sesame flavor. Use the same amount and soften the oil slightly so it blends easily. Using coconut oil will lower the protein slightly, but the macros don't change too much.

PER SERVING (1 COOKIE)
Macronutrients: Fat: 88%; Protein: 6%; Carbs: 6%
Calories: 173; Total fat: 17g; Total carbs: 2g; Fiber: 1g;
Net carbs: 1g; Sodium: 12mg; Protein: 3g

CHOCOLATE CHIP ALMOND COOKIES

SUPER QUICK

PREP TIME: 15 MINUTES | COOK TIME: 10 MINUTES

MAKES 20 COOKIES

Honestly, is there anything more comforting than chocolate chip cookies when you want a treat? My version is golden, buttery, and studded with chocolate chips—everything this iconic snack *should* be. But if you want a simple, plainer version, you could also make these almond cookies without the chips.

1 cup grass-fed butter, at room temperature

¾ cup monk fruit sweetener, granulated form

2 eggs

1 tablespoon vanilla extract

3½ cups almond flour

1 teaspoon baking soda

½ teaspoon sea salt

1½ cups keto-friendly chocolate chips, like Lily's Dark Chocolate Chips

1. **Preheat the oven.** Set the oven temperature to 350°F. Line a baking sheet with parchment paper and set it aside.

2. **Mix the wet ingredients.** In a large bowl, cream the butter and sweetener until the mixture is very fluffy, either by hand or with a hand mixer. Add the eggs and vanilla and beat until everything is well blended.

3. **Mix the dry ingredients.** In a medium bowl, stir together the almond flour, baking soda, and salt until they're well mixed together.

4. **Add the dry to the wet ingredients.** Stir the dry ingredients into the wet ingredients and mix until everything is well combined. Stir in the chocolate chips.

5. **Bake.** Drop the batter by tablespoons onto the baking sheet about 2 inches apart and flatten them down slightly. Bake the cookies for 10 minutes, or until they're golden. Repeat with any remaining dough. Transfer the cookies to a wire rack and let them cool.

6. **Store.** Store the cookies in a sealed container in the refrigerator for up to five days, or in the freezer for up to one month.

Swap: Add ½ cup chopped pecans or walnuts for a loaded, tasty cookie. Stir them in with the chips and enjoy! The extra nuts will add about 2 grams of fat and 20 calories per cookie.

PER SERVING (2 COOKIES)
Macronutrients: Fat: 92%; Protein: 6%; Carbs: 2%
Calories: 226; Total fat: 27g; Total carbs: 1g; Fiber: 1g;
Net carbs: 0g; Sodium: 134mg; Protein: 3g

RICH CHOCOLATE MUG CAKE

SUPER QUICK

PREP TIME: 5 MINUTES | COOK TIME: 1½ MINUTES

SERVES: 2

Mug cake is a trend—a sensation, even. It's also just a simple way to get a dessert fix in a couple of minutes. Even though the texture of mug cakes isn't exactly like a real baked cake, it's certainly close enough to satisfy. My recipe turns out nicely dense and chocolatey, so try putting a big scoop of whipped cream or coconut cream on top.

½ cup almond flour

2 tablespoons coconut flour

2 tablespoons cocoa powder

1¼ teaspoons baking powder

1 tablespoon monk fruit sweetener, granulated form

¼ cup melted grass-fed butter

2 eggs

½ teaspoon vanilla extract

½ cup keto-friendly chocolate chips like Lily's Dark Chocolate Chips

1. **Mix the dry ingredients.** In a medium bowl, stir together the almond flour, coconut flour, cocoa powder, baking powder, and sweetener.

2. **Finish the batter.** Stir in the melted butter, eggs, and vanilla until everything is well combined. Stir in the chocolate chips.

3. **Cook and serve.** Divide the batter between two large mugs and microwave them on high for 90 seconds, or until the cakes are cooked. Serve them immediately.

Swap: Other sugar-free chocolate chips will obviously work instead of Lily's, so use your favorite in this convenient treat. Try Hershey's Sugar Free Chocolate Chips, ChocZero chips, or chop up a ChocoPerfection bar for your recipe.

PER SERVING

Macronutrients: Fat: 78%; Protein: 11%; Carbs: 11%
Calories: 383; Total fat: 35g; Total carbs: 12g; Fiber: 7g;
Net carbs: 5g; Sodium: 104mg; Protein: 11g

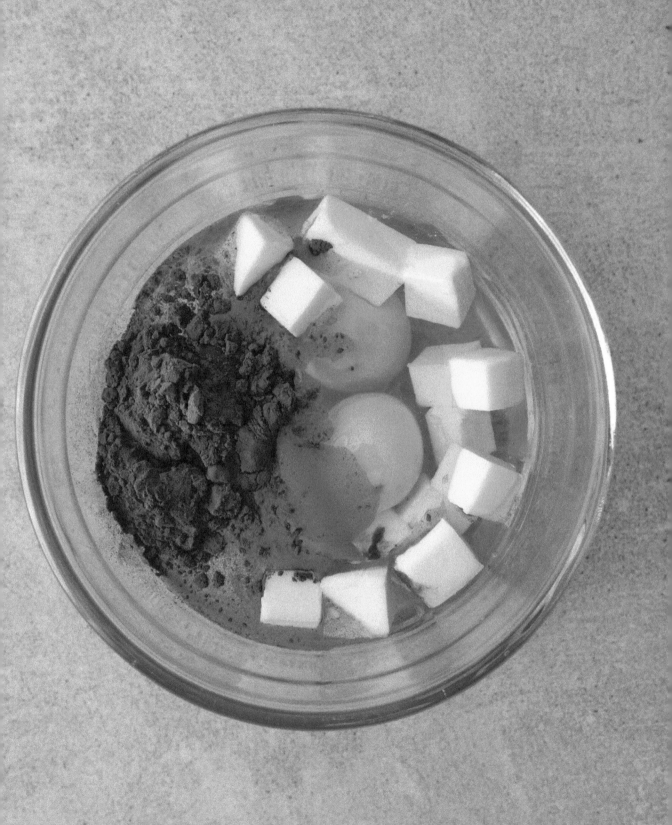

DARK CHOCOLATE FUDGE

SUPER QUICK

PREP TIME: 15 MINUTES, PLUS CHILLING TIME
MAKES 30 PIECES

Traditional fudge can be difficult to make since you need to know a lot about the different stages of sugar according to its temperature. My fudge, on the other hand, is super easy and quick, and you won't have to beat it until it feels like your arm's gonna fall off. Try flavoring it with almond extract or peppermint extract if you want to change up the flavor a little bit.

1 cup coconut oil, melted

1 cup cocoa powder

1 teaspoon vanilla extract

½ cup monk fruit sweetener, granulated form

Pinch sea salt

1. **Prepare a baking dish.** Line a 9-by-9-inch glass baking dish with plastic wrap and set it aside.

2. **Make the fudge.** Place the coconut oil, cocoa powder, vanilla, sweetener, and salt in a blender and process until the mixture is smooth and blended. Pour the mixture into the baking dish and place more plastic wrap over it.

3. **Refrigerate.** Place the fudge in the refrigerator for at least 4 hours, until it is set up and firm.

4. **Cut and store.** Remove the fudge from the baking dish, cut it into roughly 1½-inch squares and store in the freezer in a sealed container for up to one month.

Tip: Good-quality cocoa powder such as Dutch-processed cocoa powder or natural cocoa powder gives the fudge a rich, deep chocolate flavor. Try Valrhona or Guittard for stunning results.

PER SERVING (2 PIECES)
Macronutrients: Fat: 95%; Protein: 1%; Carbs: 4%
Calories: 139; Total fat: 15g; Total carbs: 3g; Fiber: 2g;
Net carbs: 1g; Sodium: 1mg; Protein: 1g

VANILLA CREAM PUDDING WITH BERRIES

SUPER QUICK

PREP TIME: 10 MINUTES, PLUS CHILLING TIME | COOK TIME: 10 MINUTES

SERVES: 6

This is a classic, creamy cooked pudding that you can serve for dessert, but it also works as a nice breakfast, especially for kids. The coconut milk can be combined with almond milk in equal amounts if you want a lighter version. And if you're going for a festive look, spoon the pudding into glasses in layers with whipped cream. That'll make really gorgeous parfaits you can top with berries.

3 cups coconut milk

⅓ cup monk fruit sweetener, granulated form

¼ cup arrowroot flour

1 egg

1 tablespoon coconut oil

1 tablespoon pure vanilla extract

1 cup fresh blueberries

1. **Cook the base.** In a large saucepan, whisk together the coconut milk, sweetener, and arrowroot. Bring the mixture to a boil then reduce the heat to low, whisking constantly, until the pudding is thick, about 5 minutes. Whisk the egg into the pudding and cook, while still whisking, for about 30 seconds.

2. **Add the remaining ingredients.** Whisk the coconut oil and vanilla into the pudding until it's smooth.

3. **Cool.** Transfer the pudding to a medium bowl and cover it with plastic wrap, pressing the wrap down to the surface of the pudding, then place it in the refrigerator to cool completely, about 2 hours.

4. **Serve.** Spoon the pudding into bowls and top with the blueberries.

Swap: If you want a colorful topping or fewer carbs, try swapping in other berries like strawberries, blackberries, or raspberries.

PER SERVING

Macronutrients: Fat: 80%; Protein: 7%; Carbs: 13%
Calories: 286; Total fat: 27g; Total carbs: 9g; Fiber: 2g;
Net carbs: 7g; Sodium: 28mg; Protein: 3g

TIRAMISU

FULL GUIDO

PREP TIME: 30 MINUTES, PLUS CHILLING TIME | COOK TIME: 25 MINUTES
SERVES: 4

This is my all-time favorite dessert. When we filmed *Jersey Shore* in Italy, we went to Tuscany and the whole cast took this tiramisu-baking class from an expert Italian woman. What I learned in that class allowed me to create this recipe, which is delicious. In fact, my aunt Antonella (aka Zia Lella) is famous for her tiramisu, and at holiday parties now, we both make our versions and go head-to-head with taste tests to determine whose is better. (Mine.)

FOR THE LADY FINGERS

- 1 cup almond flour
- 1 teaspoon baking powder
- 3 large eggs, yolks and whites separated
- ½ cup monk fruit sweetener, granulated form
- 1 teaspoon vanilla extract

TO MAKE THE LADY FINGERS

1. **Preheat the oven.** Set the oven temperature to 350°F. Line a baking sheet with parchment paper and set it aside. Fit a large pastry bag with a ½-inch tip.

2. **Mix the dry ingredients.** In a small bowl, stir together the almond flour and baking powder.

3. **Beat the yolks.** In a medium bowl, beat the egg yolks together with the sweetener until the yolks are pale yellow, about 6 minutes. Set them aside.

4. **Beat the whites.** In another medium bowl, beat the egg whites until soft peaks form. Fold the whites into the egg yolks, keeping as much volume as possible. Fold in the vanilla.

5. **Add the dry ingredients.** Fold the dry ingredients into the egg-white mixture and then spoon the batter into a piping bag (if you don't have one, you can use a plastic bag with one corner snipped off).

6. **Pipe the lady fingers and bake.** Pipe the lady fingers into 3-inch lines on the baking sheet, about 16 in total. Bake them for about 15 minutes, until they're firm to the touch. Transfer them to a wire rack and let them cool.

FOR THE TIRAMISU

3 egg yolks

¼ cup monk fruit sweetener, granulated form

½ cup mascarpone cheese, at room temperature

¾ cup heavy (whipping) cream

½ cup cold espresso, made from powder

1 teaspoon cocoa powder, for dusting

TO MAKE THE TIRAMISU

1. **Beat the yolks.** Place a large bowl over a medium pot of gently simmering water. Add the egg yolks and sweetener to the bowl and beat constantly until the yolks are thick and pale yellow, about 10 minutes. Remove the bowl from the heat and let the yolks cool for 10 minutes.

2. **Mix in the mascarpone cheese.** Beat the mascarpone into the yolks until well blended.

3. **Beat the cream.** In a medium bowl, beat the cream until stiff peaks form. Fold the whipped cream into the mascarpone mixture and set it aside.

4. **Assemble the tiramisu.** Dip eight lady fingers into the espresso and arrange two each in four bowls. Divide half of the mascarpone mixture between the bowls, spreading it over the lady fingers. Dip the remaining eight lady fingers in the espresso and arrange two per bowl on top of the mascarpone mixture. Divide the remaining mascarpone mixture between the bowls, spread it over the lady fingers, and smooth the tops.

CONTINUED ▶

5. **Chill.** Refrigerate the individual tiramisus over-night, covered with plastic wrap.

6. **Serve.** Dust the tiramisus with the cocoa and serve them chilled.

Tip: In order to make this recipe slightly less labor intensive, make the lady fingers ahead and store them in a covered container in the refrigerator for up to one week. The best part is, even if they harden up a bit it doesn't matter because you'll be soaking them in espresso.

Swap: You can use a light keto sponge cake instead of the lady fingers to save time, but if you do, drizzle the espresso over it instead of dipping the whole thing because if you dip it, the cake will fall apart.

PER SERVING
Macronutrients: Fat: 85%; Protein: 11%; Carbs: 4%
Calories: 344; Total fat: 33g; Total carbs: 3g; Fiber: 1g;
Net carbs: 2g; Sodium: 84mg; Protein: 10g

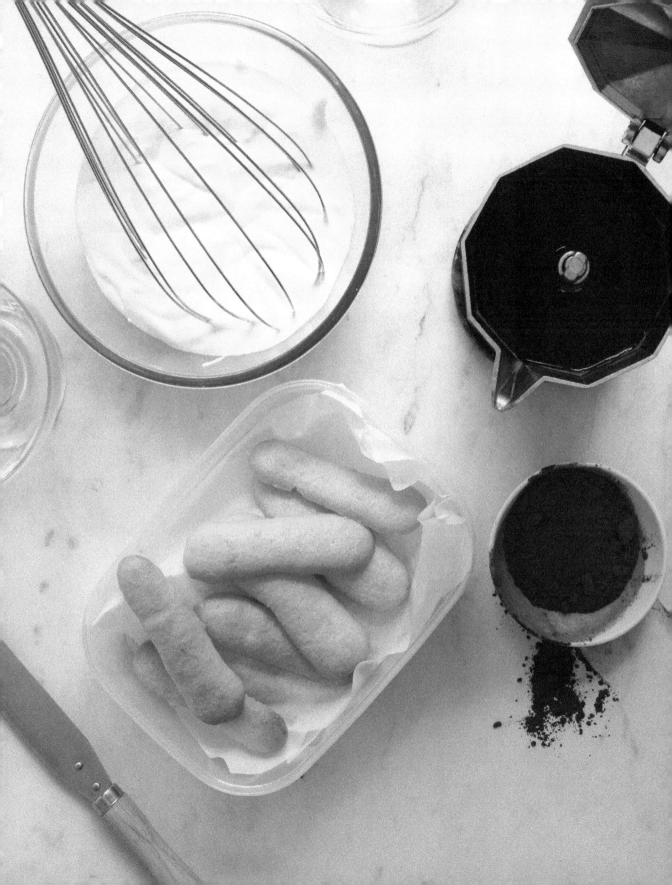

FLUFFY COCONUT MOUSSE

SUPER QUICK

PREP TIME: 15 MINUTES, PLUS CHILLING TIME | COOK TIME: 5 MINUTES
SERVES: 4

Mousse has this nice light texture that makes it the perfect end to a good meal like grilled steak served outside on a warm summer night. Gelatin might seem like an intimidating ingredient, but it's easy to use as long as you follow the instructions and let it soften. For this recipe, either granulated gelatin or gelatin sheets will work.

¼ cup cold water

2 teaspoons granulated gelatin

1 cup coconut milk

3 egg yolks

½ cup monk fruit sweetener, granulated form

1 cup heavy (whipping) cream

1. **Prepare the gelatin.** Pour the cold water into a small bowl, sprinkle the gelatin on top, and set it aside for 10 minutes.

2. **Heat the coconut milk.** Place a small saucepan over medium heat and pour in the coconut milk. Bring the coconut milk to a boil then remove the pan from the heat.

3. **Thicken the base.** Whisk the eggs and sweetener in a medium bowl. Pour the coconut milk into the yolks and whisk it to blend. Pour the yolk mixture back into the saucepan and place it over medium heat. Whisk until the base thickens, about 5 minutes. Remove the pan from the heat and whisk in the gelatin mixture.

4. **Cool.** Transfer the mixture to a medium bowl and cool it completely in the refrigerator, about 1 hour.

5. **Make the mousse.** When the coconut milk mixture is cool, whisk the cream in a large bowl until it's thick and fluffy, about 3 minutes. Fold the whipped cream into the coconut mixture until the mousse is well combined and fluffy.

6. **Serve.** Divide the mousse between four bowls and serve it immediately.

Tip: You can increase the coconut taste by mixing in a teaspoon of coconut extract and sprinkling the top with a toasted coconut garnish. Use a light hand with the topping because too much will ruin the melt-in-your-mouth texture.

Swap: Make it chocolate! Add 2 tablespoons of cocoa powder when heating the coconut milk, stirring well to remove any lumps, and increase the sweetener to ¾ cup. This chocolate mousse also works well as frosting for a keto cake.

PER SERVING
Macronutrients: Fat: 88%; Protein: 8%; Carbs: 4%
Calories: 261; Total fat: 27g; Total carbs: 3g; Fiber: 0g;
Net carbs: 3g; Sodium: 28mg; Protein: 5g

NEW YORK CHEESECAKE

FULL GUIDO

PREP TIME: 15 MINUTES | COOK TIME: 1 HOUR, 25 MINUTES
SERVES: 12

Cheesecake is almost like a religion to some people. It's decadent, it's rich, and the texture is nice and creamy. New York cheesecake is the ultimate accomplishment because it's not hiding behind toppings, chocolate, or any flavorings—it's perfect in its plainness. That being said, of course you *can* top this with something if you want, like fresh berries or a little whipped cream.

FOR THE CRUST

1½ cups almond flour

3 tablespoons monk fruit sweetener, granulated form

⅓ cup melted grass-fed butter

FOR THE FILLING

2½ pounds cream cheese, at room temperature

1¼ cups monk fruit sweetener, granulated form

3 tablespoons arrowroot

¼ teaspoon sea salt

5 eggs, lightly beaten

2 egg yolks

2 teaspoons vanilla extract

Zest of ½ lemon

½ cup heavy (whipping) cream

TO MAKE THE CRUST

1. **Preheat the oven.** Set the oven temperature to 350°F.

2. **Mix the crust ingredients.** In a medium bowl, stir together the almond flour, sweetener, and melted butter until the ingredients hold together when pressed. Press the crumbs into the bottom of a 10-inch springform pan.

3. **Chill and bake.** Chill the crust in the freezer for 10 minutes. Transfer it to the oven and bake it for 10 minutes. Cool the crust completely before filling.

TO MAKE THE FILLING

1. **Change the oven temperature.** Increase the oven temperature to 450°F.

2. **Beat the cream cheese.** In a large bowl, beat the cream cheese with an electric mixer until it's very light and fluffy, scraping down the sides several times with a spatula.

3. **Add the dry ingredients.** Beat in the sweetener, arrowroot, and salt until very smooth, scraping down the sides at least once.

4. **Beat in the wet ingredients.** Beat in the eggs and egg yolks one at a time, scraping down the sides of the bowl between each addition. Beat in the vanilla and lemon zest. Add the cream, beating until just blended.

5. **Pour and bake.** Pour the filling into the pre-baked crust and bake it for 15 minutes. Reduce the oven temperature to 200°F and bake for 1 hour.

6. **Cool.** Turn the oven off and, without opening the oven door, let the cheesecake cool in the oven for 1 hour. Then transfer the cheesecake to a countertop, run a knife around the edge of the cheesecake, and let it cool to room temperature. Chill it in the refrigerator for at least 4 to 6 hours.

7. **Serve.** Cut the cheesecake into 12 slices and serve.

Tip: Make sure you beat the cream cheese completely smooth before adding any of the other ingredients because that is your only chance to get out all the lumps.

PER SERVING
Macronutrients: Fat: 87%; Protein: 9%; Carbs: 4%
Calories: 440; Total fat: 43g; Total carbs: 5g; Fiber: 0g;
Net carbs: 5g; Sodium: 337mg; Protein: 9g

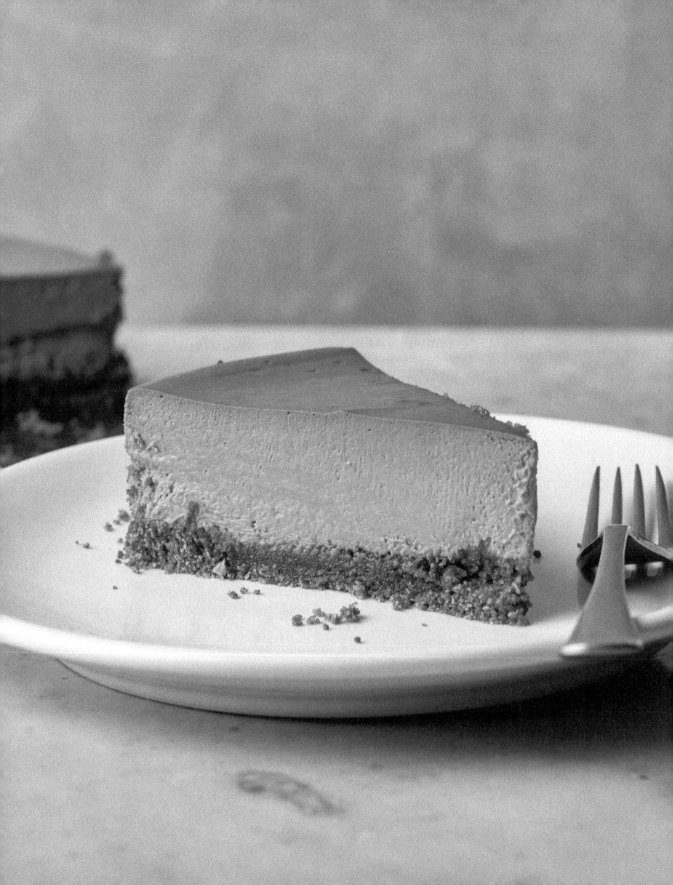

CHOCOLATE CHEESECAKE WITH TOASTED ALMOND CRUST

FULL GUIDO

PREP TIME: 15 MINUTES | COOK TIME: 1 HOUR, 20 MINUTES

SERVES: 10

This is a glorious dessert, with a dense, fudgy texture through the middle and a really powerful chocolate flavor thanks to the double chocolate impact of the crust and the base. You might think it's underdone at first, but let it cool completely before you cut it and you won't be disappointed. Make sure not to open the oven during the baking or cooling time, because a burst of cooler air can make the cheesecake crack.

FOR THE CRUST

1½ cups almond flour

4 tablespoons monk fruit sweetener, granulated form

1 tablespoon cocoa powder

⅓ cup melted grass-fed butter

FOR THE FILLING

1½ pounds cream cheese, softened

¾ cup monk fruit sweetener, granulated form

3 eggs, beaten

1 teaspoon vanilla extract

½ teaspoon almond extract (optional)

5 ounces keto-friendly chocolate chips like Lily's Dark Chocolate Chips, melted and cooled

1 cup sour cream

TO MAKE THE CRUST

1. **Preheat the oven.** Set the oven temperature to 350°F.

2. **Mix the crust ingredients.** In a medium bowl, stir together the almond flour, sweetener, cocoa powder, and melted butter until the ingredients hold together when pressed. Press the crumbs into the bottom of a 10-inch springform pan and 1 inch up the sides.

3. **Chill and bake.** Chill the crust in the freezer for 10 minutes. Transfer it to the oven and bake it for 10 minutes. Cool the crust completely before filling.

TO MAKE THE FILLING

1. **Change the oven temperature.** Reduce the oven temperature to 275°F.

2. **Mix the cheesecake base.** In a large bowl, beat the cream cheese until very light and fluffy, scraping down the sides with a spatula at least once. Beat in the sweetener until the mixture is smooth, scraping down the sides of the bowl.

CONTINUED

3. **Add the eggs.** Beat in the eggs one at a time, scraping down the sides of the bowl occasionally and then beat in the vanilla extract and almond extract (if using).

4. **Add the remaining ingredients.** Beat in the melted chocolate and sour cream until the filling is well blended, scraping down the sides of the bowl.

5. **Bake.** Pour the filling into the prebaked crust and bake it for 1 hour and 10 minutes. Turn off the oven and cool the cheesecake in the closed oven until it reaches room temperature.

6. **Chill.** Chill the cheesecake in the refrigerator for at least 4 to 6 hours.

7. **Serve.** Cut the cheesecake into 10 slices and serve.

Tip: Make sure the ingredients are all at a similar temperature, including letting the melted chocolate cool so it doesn't go grainy when put into a cold base. You want a smooth cheesecake batter to create the perfect texture.

PER SERVING
Macronutrients: Fat: 88%; Protein: 8%; Carbs: 4%
Calories: 408; Total fat: 40g; Total carbs: 4g; Fiber: 0g;
Net carbs: 4g; Sodium: 258mg; Protein: 8g

LEMON COCONUT TRUFFLES

SUPER QUICK

PREP TIME: 30 MINUTES

MAKES 16 TRUFFLES

Truffles are elegant and sound expensive—they make me think of French patisseries or fancy restaurants. My recipe might seem a little strange because traditional chocolate truffles are formed from chocolate ganache, but trust me, these turn out delicious. The base is smooth, and then the tartness of the lemon does a beautiful job offsetting the sweetener. Make sure to mince the lemon zest very well so there aren't any long strings of it in the truffles.

3 cups shredded unsweetened coconut, divided

½ cup pecans

2 tablespoons coconut oil

Zest and juice of 1 lemon

½ cup monk fruit sweetener, granulated form

Pinch sea salt

1. **Make the truffle base.** Put 2 cups of the coconut and the pecans in a food processor and pulse until the mixture looks like a paste, about 5 minutes.

2. **Add the remaining ingredients.** Add the coconut oil, lemon zest, lemon juice, sweetener, and salt to the processor and pulse until the mixture forms a big ball, about 2 minutes.

3. **Form the truffles.** Scoop the mixture out with a tablespoon and roll it into 16 balls. Roll the truffles in the remaining 1 cup of coconut.

4. **Store.** Store the truffles in a sealed container in the refrigerator for up to one week or in the freezer for up to one month.

Swap: Try 2 limes instead of 1 lemon, or use one of each for a complex flavor that sparks your taste buds.

PER SERVING (1 TRUFFLE)
Macronutrients: Fat: 84%; Protein: 4%; Carbs: 12%
Calories: 160; Total fat: 16g; Total carbs: 5g; Fiber: 3g;
Net carbs: 2g; Sodium: 24mg; Protein: 2g

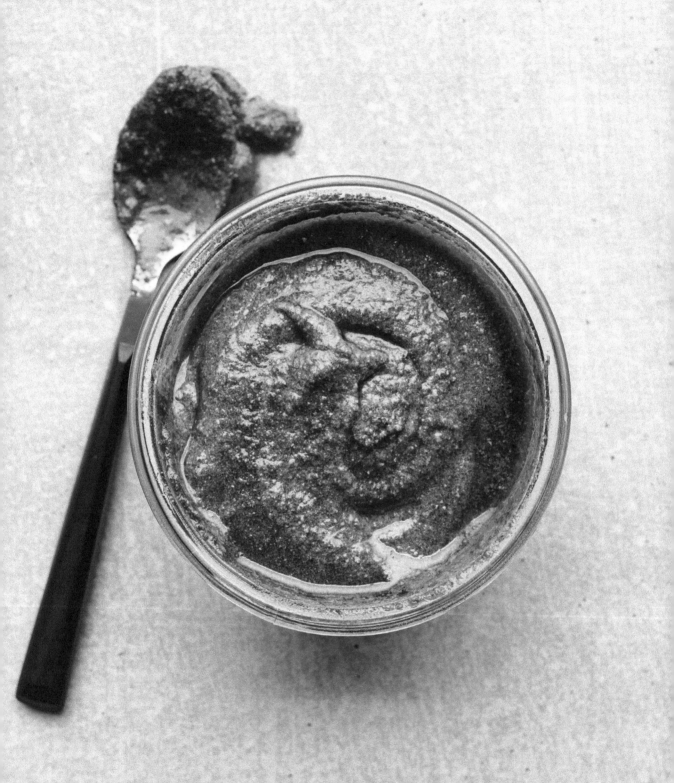

Staples and Drinks

It's possible to get burnt out if you're eating the same foods on keto all the time. That's why I made these recipes to help you switch things up. A new sauce, a new dressing, or even a new twist on the drinks you're having every day can make what you're eating feel brand-new again.

SPINACH BASIL PESTO

SUPER QUICK | FULL GUIDO
PREP TIME: 10 MINUTES
MAKES 2 CUPS

Pesto is one of those condiments that can be used in a huge number of dishes and combined with almost any ingredient. Things like simple vegetable noodles, chicken, beef, fish, vegetables, dips, and sauces can all benefit from pesto. You can even stir it into scrambled eggs or soup for a flavor boost—really, the only limit is your imagination.

2 cups fresh spinach

1 cup fresh basil leaves

3 garlic cloves, smashed

¼ cup pecans

¼ cup grated
   Parmesan cheese

½ cup good-quality
   olive oil

Sea salt, for seasoning

Freshly ground black
   pepper, for seasoning

1. **Blend the base.** Put the spinach, basil, garlic, pecans, and Parmesan in a blender and pulse until the mixture is finely chopped, scraping down the sides of the blender once.

2. **Finish the pesto.** While the blender is running, pour in the olive oil in a thin stream and blend until the pesto is smooth. Season it with salt and pepper.

3. **Store.** Store in a sealed container in the refrigerator for up to one week.

Swap: Pesto comes in many variations because this delectable creation is versatile. Try kale, basil, or cilantro in place of the spinach in the same amount.

PER SERVING (2 TABLESPOONS)
Macronutrients: Fat: 89%; Protein: 6%; Carbs: 5%
Calories: 60; Total fat: 6g; Total carbs: 1g; Fiber: 0g;
Net carbs: 1g; Sodium: 27mg; Protein: 1g

CREAMY ALFREDO SAUCE

SUPER QUICK | FULL GUIDO
PREP TIME: 10 MINUTES | COOK TIME: 10 MINUTES
SERVES: 6

Alfredo sauce is one of the richest, most decadent creations ever to be served over noodles. I guess it's no surprise that it's an American creation and isn't really served in Italy because over there, cream isn't a common thing to add to sauce. Even so, my mom made this all the time, so growing up, my favorite pasta dish was fettuccine Alfredo. These days, I make my own sauce, and like to spoon it over grilled chicken, zucchini noodles, roasted cauliflower, or even drizzle it over meatballs.

¼ cup grass-fed butter

1 cup cream cheese

1½ cups heavy (whip-ping) cream

2 teaspoons minced garlic

¼ teaspoon salt

¼ teaspoon freshly ground black pepper

1 cup grated Parmesan cheese

1. **Make the sauce.** In a medium saucepan over medium heat, stir together the butter, cream cheese, and cream. Cook, whisking until the sauce is smooth and the butter and cheese are melted. Add the garlic, salt, and pepper and whisk until well blended. Whisk in the Parmesan.

2. **Simmer.** Bring the sauce to a simmer and cook until it is slightly thickened, about 5 minutes.

3. **Store.** Cool the sauce completely and store in a sealed container in the refrigerator for up to three days.

Swap: Use a soft goat cheese instead of cream cheese for a richer taste and thicker, creamier texture.

PER SERVING
Macronutrients: Fat: 88%; Protein: 9%; Carbs: 3%
Calories: 478; Total fat: 48g; Total carbs: 4g; Fiber: 0g;
Net carbs: 4g; Sodium: 552mg; Protein: 10g

TRADITIONAL MEAT SAUCE

FULL GUIDO

PREP TIME: 15 MINUTES | COOK TIME: 40 MINUTES

SERVES: 4

This isn't a classic Bolognese sauce because it doesn't include pork and it isn't simmered for hours on the stove. It's a simpler, speedier version. You can use fresh tomatoes instead of canned, if so, add some beef stock to replace the juices from the canned ones. And definitely adjust the herbs and garlic for your own palate. You can use this on whatever you eat—I like to pour it over a bowl of zucchini noodles.

2 tablespoons good-quality olive oil

1 pound grass-fed ground beef

1 onion, chopped

2 celery stalks, chopped

2 tablespoons minced garlic

1 (28-ounce) can sodium-free diced tomatoes

¼ cup red wine

¼ cup tomato paste

2 teaspoons dried oregano

2 teaspoons dried basil

1 teaspoon dried parsley

½ teaspoon sea salt

¼ teaspoon red pepper flakes

1. **Brown the beef.** In a large pot over medium-high heat, warm the olive oil. Brown the ground beef, stirring it occasionally, until it's cooked through, about 6 minutes.

2. **Sauté the vegetables.** Stir in the onion, celery, and garlic and sauté them until they've softened, about 3 minutes.

3. **Add the rest of the ingredients.** Stir in the tomatoes, red wine, tomato paste, oregano, basil, parsley, salt, and red pepper flakes.

4. **Cook the sauce.** Bring the sauce to a boil, then reduce the heat to low and simmer it for 25 to 30 minutes, stirring occasionally.

5. **Store.** Cool the sauce completely and store in a sealed container in the refrigerator for up to four days or freeze for up to one month.

Swap: Chicken, pork, bison, and lamb can be substituted for the beef. Prepare the recipe exactly the same and use the same amount as the beef.

PER SERVING

Macronutrients: Fat: 70%; Protein: 20%; Carbs: 10%

Calories: 457; Total fat: 35g; Total carbs: 13g; Fiber: 5g;

Net carbs: 8g; Sodium: 345mg; Protein: 21g

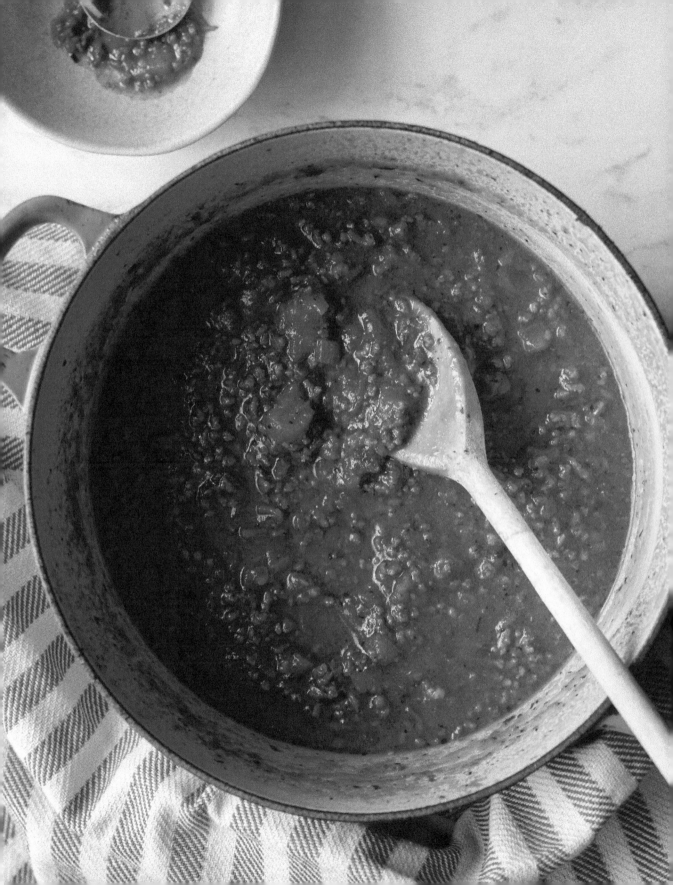

EASY KETO GRAVY

SUPER QUICK

PREP TIME: 5 MINUTES | COOK TIME: 20 MINUTES

SERVES: 4

Among Italian Americans, there's on ongoing debate about what the word "gravy" refers to. Some people say that the red stuff made from tomatoes is "gravy," but real Italians know that's wrong—the red stuff is "sauce" and the brown stuff is "gravy." My family is off-the-boat Sicilian and would never confuse the two, so in honor of them, this recipe is officially considered gravy. Whatever you decide to call it, this stuff is delicious. You can easily make it with pan drippings from turkey, chicken, or roasts, so whenever possible, use that instead of stocks.

¼ cup grass-fed butter, divided

½ onion, finely chopped

1 teaspoon minced garlic

2 cups Beef Bone Broth (page 236) or Chicken Bone Broth (page 238)

2 large egg yolks

Sea salt, for seasoning

Freshly ground black pepper, for seasoning

1. **Sauté the aromatics.** In a medium saucepan over medium heat, melt 1 tablespoon of the butter. Add the onion and garlic and sauté until they've softened, about 3 minutes.

2. **Cook the broth.** Stir in the broth and bring it to a boil, then reduce the heat to low and simmer until the liquid is slightly thickened, about 10 minutes.

3. **Blend.** Transfer the mixture to a blender and blend until it's smooth. Pour it back into the saucepan, this time over low heat.

4. **Add the egg yolks.** Whisk the egg yolks in a small bowl. Whisk about ¼ cup of the hot liquid into the yolks, then pour this mixture into the broth, whisking constantly.

5. **Add the butter.** While the broth is simmering and while whisking constantly, add the remaining butter and whisk until it's melted and the gravy is smooth and thick, about 4 minutes.

6. Serve. Serve immediately with salt and pepper or cool then store in the refrigerator in a sealed container for up to three days.

Tip: The flavor of this gravy depends entirely on the quality of the stock used, so make sure it has a strong taste and is not too salty. The best choice is homemade, but you can use a low-sodium pur-chased broth as well.

PER SERVING
Macronutrients: Fat: 82%; Protein: 11%; Carbs: 7%
Calories: 147; Total fat: 14g; Total carbs: 3g; Fiber: 0g;
Net carbs: 3g; Sodium: 157mg; Protein: 4g

CLASSIC AIOLI

SUPER QUICK | FULL GUIDO
PREP TIME: 10 MINUTES
SERVES: 8

Aioli is just a word that means garlic mayonnaise. It comes from French, where it combines the words for garlic and oil. The best way to make aioli is to use both olive oil and canola oil to create a milder taste, but my recipe only uses olive oil to keep that unhealthy canola oil as far away from our bodies as possible. But you should try to track down a milder, fruitier olive oil to offset the missing canola oil, and don't use extra-virgin olive oil, because it will make your mixture split.

1 large egg

2 teaspoons Dijon mustard

1½ teaspoons minced garlic

1 cup olive oil

1 tablespoon freshly squeezed lemon juice

Sea salt, for seasoning

1. **Combine the base.** In a medium bowl, whisk together the egg, mustard, and garlic until they're well blended, about 2 minutes.

2. **Add the oil.** Slowly add the olive oil in a thin, continuous stream, whisking constantly until the aioli is thick. Whisk in the lemon juice and season the aioli with salt.

3. **Store.** Store the aioli in an airtight container in the refrigerator for up to four days.

Tip: Roast the garlic before adding it in. Put peeled garlic cloves in an oven-safe skillet and drizzle them with olive oil. Cover the skillet with foil and bake at 350°F for about 15 minutes, or until the garlic is golden brown and softened. Add 1 roasted garlic clove instead of the minced garlic.

Swap: Make it fancy by adding some truffle oil to this, too.

PER SERVING (1 TABLESPOON)
Macronutrients: Fat: 98%; Protein: 1%; Carbs: 1%
Calories: 124; Total fat: 14g; Total carbs: 0g; Fiber: 0g;
Net carbs: 0g; Sodium: 12mg; Protein: 0g

AVOCADO BUTTERMILK DRESSING

SUPER QUICK

PREP TIME: 10 MINUTES

MAKES 1½ CUPS

This is a really delicious dressing. It's pale green and looks great on top of a spring salad or drizzled on grilled vegetables. Buttermilk is the liquid that's left behind after churning butter out of cultured cream, so it's pretty low in fat, which is why I added coconut milk to the mix. You can use a whole avocado if you want to end up with a thicker dressing and a stronger fruit flavor.

¼ cup buttermilk

¼ cup coconut milk

½ avocado

2 tablespoons chopped fresh dill

1 tablespoon freshly squeezed lemon juice

1 teaspoon minced garlic

½ teaspoon sweet paprika

Sea salt, for seasoning

Freshly ground black pepper, for seasoning

1. **Make the dressing.** Put the buttermilk, coconut milk, avocado, dill, lemon juice, garlic, and sweet paprika in a blender and blend until the dressing is very smooth. Season it with salt and pepper.

2. **Store.** Store the dressing in a sealed container in the refrigerator for up to five days.

Swap: If you don't have buttermilk, mix heavy cream with a teaspoon of white vinegar to create a tangy substitution. The heavy cream will also add more fat to the recipe.

PER SERVING (2 TABLESPOONS)
Macronutrients: Fat: 74%; Protein: 8%; Carbs: 18%
Calories: 22; Total fat: 2g; Total carbs: 1g; Fiber: 0g;
Net carbs: 1g; Sodium: 32mg; Protein: 0g

HOMEMADE RANCH DRESSING

SUPER QUICK
PREP TIME: 5 MINUTES
MAKES 2 CUPS

Ranch dressing is a staple in many homes. You might be wondering why you'd make it from scratch when there are so many great products in grocery stores. It's because those are usually high in carbs due to all the added sugars and thickeners. When you make your own, you can leave out those ingredients. Use this dressing on your salads, as a dip, or even drizzled over chicken and fish.

¾ cup coconut milk

½ cup buttermilk

¼ cup plain Greek yogurt

¼ cup minced onion

2 tablespoons chopped fresh parsley

2 tablespoons chopped fresh chives

1 tablespoon chopped fresh dill

Sea salt, for seasoning

Fresh ground black pepper, for seasoning

1. **Make the dressing.** In a medium bowl, whisk together the coconut milk, buttermilk, yogurt, onion, parsley, chives, and dill. Season the dressing with salt and pepper.

2. **Store.** Store the dressing in a sealed container in the refrigerator for up to one week.

Tip: You can grow your own fresh herbs easily in your kitchen or on a window ledge. Chives are particularly easy, and you can snip them off when you need them and the plant will continue to grow.

PER SERVING
Macronutrients: Fat: 75%; Protein: 10%; Carbs: 15%
Calories: 44; Total fat: 4g; Total carbs: 1g; Fiber: 0g;
Net carbs: 1g; Sodium: 15mg; Protein: 1g

COCONUT OIL SPIKED GREEN TEA

SUPER QUICK

PREP TIME: 1 MINUTE | COOK TIME: 5 MINUTES

SERVES: 1

You might've tried adding fat to coffee, but trust me, adding fat to tea can be just as delicious if you do it right. And the coconut oil doesn't make your tea taste oily, as long as you drink it hot. If you like the taste of honey more than the sweetener, you can use a little of that instead (even though some stricter keto-ers might shake their heads).

1 packet (0.8 gram) Monk Fruit in the Raw sweetener

1 tablespoon coconut oil

Juice of 1 lime

1 green tea bag

Water, heated to just boiling

1. **Mix.** In a large mug, stir together the sweetener, coconut oil, and lime juice.

2. **Steep.** Add the tea bag and enough water to fill the mug. Let the tea steep for 3 minutes.

3. **Serve.** Remove the tea bag, stir to blend, and serve immediately.

Swap: Green tea is a healthy option, but any tea can be enhanced by coconut oil and a bit of sweetener. I like herbal tea such as hibiscus, lemon, or even spiced apple tea.

PER SERVING
Macronutrients: Fat: 92%; Protein: 0%; Carbs: 8%
Calories: 127; Total fat: 14g; Total carbs: 4g; Fiber: 0g;
Net carbs: 4g; Sodium: 1mg; Protein: 0g

CAFÉ STYLE FATTY COFFEE

SUPER QUICK

PREP TIME: 2 MINUTES

SERVES: 1

This is your base coffee. It's simple, just a little bit sweet, and it's got a satisfying hint of cinnamon, like something a high-end barista would make. Adding butter to your coffee isn't just a keto thing, by the way—different cultures have been doing it for centuries, like ones in the Himalayas and Ethiopia. The theory is that the butter slows the uptake of caffeine to deliver energy to you throughout the day.

1 cup freshly brewed coffee

2 teaspoons coconut oil or MCT oil

1 teaspoon grass-fed butter

1 packet (0.8 gram) Monk Fruit in the Raw sweetener

Ground cinnamon, for garnish

1. **Blend.** Place the freshly brewed coffee, coconut oil, butter, and sweetener in a blender and pulse until it's creamy and a bit foamy.

2. **Serve.** Pour the coffee into a mug and top with a sprinkle of cinnamon. Serve it immediately.

Tip: You can just stir the oil into the coffee, but you won't get the amazing creamy texture the blender produces. If you have a stick blender, that will work perfectly.

PER SERVING
Macronutrients: Fat: 98%; Protein: 1%; Carbs: 1%
Calories: 117; Total fat: 13g; Total carbs: 1g; Fiber: 0g;
Net carbs: 1g; Sodium: 12mg; Protein: 0g

CHOCOLATE MINT FATTY COFFEE

SUPER QUICK

PREP TIME: 3 MINUTES

SERVES: 1

If you want to impress someone when you wake up together in the morning, try this. It's a really decadent concoction. The peppermint and chocolate combo in this reminds me of Christmas, but I like to make it year-round because it's so good.

1 cup freshly brewed coffee

2 tablespoons heavy (whipping) cream

2 teaspoons coconut oil or MCT oil

2 teaspoons cocoa powder

1 teaspoon grass-fed butter

½ teaspoon peppermint extract

1 packet (0.8 gram) Monk Fruit in the Raw sweetener

1. **Blend.** Put the coffee, cream, coconut oil, cocoa powder, butter, peppermint extract, and sweetener in a blender and pulse until it's creamy and slightly frothy.

2. **Serve.** Pour the coffee into a mug and serve.

Tip: Go easy on the peppermint extract since you're adding 1 gram of carbs per teaspoon.

Swap: Peppermint and chocolate are a classic combination, but other flavors can be added for variation. Try hazelnut, maple, vanilla, banana, and almond extracts in the same amount as the peppermint.

PER SERVING
Macronutrients: Fat: 92%; Protein: 2%; Carbs: 3%
Calories: 230; Total fat: 24g; Total carbs: 3g; Fiber: 2g;
Net carbs: 1g; Sodium: 43mg; Protein: 1g

BEEF BONE BROTH

FULL GUIDO

PREP TIME: 15 MINUTES | COOK TIME: 7 HOURS

MAKES 10 CUPS

Beef bone broth is a culinary trend for people who take their health seriously, because it's low-calorie and packed with lots of important minerals and nutrients. It can speed healing, boost your immune system, and help eliminate inflammation in the body. Don't skip the apple cider vinegar in this recipe—it leeches minerals from the bones you're cooking to maximize the health benefits of this recipe.

3 pounds beef bones (such as ribs, beef marrow, knuckles)

3 carrots, chopped into 1-inch pieces

3 celery stalks, cut into large chunks

1 onion, peeled and quartered

6 garlic cloves, lightly crushed

8 black peppercorns

3 bay leaves

3 tablespoons apple cider vinegar

1. **Preheat the oven.** Set the oven temperature to 350°F.

2. **Roast the bones.** Place the beef bones in a large roasting pan and roast them for 1 hour.

3. **Combine the ingredients.** Transfer the bones to a large stockpot. Add the carrots, celery, onion, garlic, peppercorns, and bay leaves and stir to mix. Add enough water to cover the bones by about 5 inches. Stir in the apple cider vinegar.

4. **Cook the bone broth.** Put the stockpot over high heat and bring the water to a boil, then reduce the heat to low, cover the pot, and simmer gently for 4 to 6 hours, skimming off any foam that forms.

5. **Cool and strain.** Let the broth cool for 30 minutes, then use tongs to remove the larger bones. Strain the stock into a large bowl and throw out the leftover vegetables and bones.

6. **Store.** Pour the broth into clean jars or containers and let it cool. Seal the jars and refrigerate for up to five days or freeze for up to two months.

Tip: Beef bones are readily available in most grocery stores or local butchers. They are often in the freezer section or behind the counter, so talk to your butcher if you don't see them.

PER SERVING
Macronutrients: Fat: 56%; Protein: 38%; Carbs: 6%
Calories: 64; Total fat: 4g; Total carbs: 1g; Fiber: 0g;
Net carbs: 1g; Sodium: 46mg; Protein: 6g

CHICKEN BONE BROTH

FULL GUIDO

PREP TIME: 15 MINUTES | COOK TIME: 7 HOURS

MAKES 10 CUPS

How many times in your life have you heard that chicken soup can cure the common cold? They even made a whole line of books about how it can cure the *soul*. And there actually might be some science behind the health aspects of chicken stock. Chicken contains cysteine, which is a natural amino acid that can thin the congestion in your lungs and make it easier to breathe. But don't wait until you're sick to make my chicken bone broth, which you can sip throughout the whole day even when you feel totally healthy.

2 chicken carcasses

4 celery stalks with leaves, cut into 2-inch chunks

2 carrots, cut into 2-inch chunks

1 onion, peeled and quartered

6 garlic cloves, lightly crushed

8 black peppercorns

3 thyme sprigs

3 bay leaves

3 tablespoons apple cider vinegar

1. **Preheat the oven.** Set the oven temperature to 350°F.

2. **Roast the bones.** Place the chicken carcasses in a large roasting pan and roast for 1 hour.

3. **Combine the ingredients.** Transfer the carcasses to a large stockpot. Add the celery, carrots, onion, garlic, peppercorns, thyme sprigs, and bay leaves and stir to mix. Add enough water to cover the ingredients by about 4 inches. Stir in the apple cider vinegar.

4. **Cook the broth.** Place the stockpot over high heat and bring the water to a boil, then reduce the heat to low, cover the pot, and simmer gently for 4 to 6 hours, skimming off any foam that forms.

5. **Cool and strain.** Let the broth cool for 30 minutes and then use tongs to remove the larger bones. Strain the stock into a large bowl and throw out the leftover vegetables and bones.

6. **Store.** Pour the broth into clean jars or containers and let it cool. Seal the jars and refrigerate for up to five days or freeze for up to two months.

Tip: Save the carcasses of any roast chickens you prepare for dinner and store them in a plastic bag in the freezer for up to two months. You will then have them on hand to make this delicious broth.

PER SERVING
Macronutrients: Fat: 0%; Protein: 88%; Carbs: 12%
Calories: 41; Total fat: 0g; Total carbs: 1g; Fiber: 0g; **Net carbs:** 1g; Sodium: 34mg; Protein: 9g

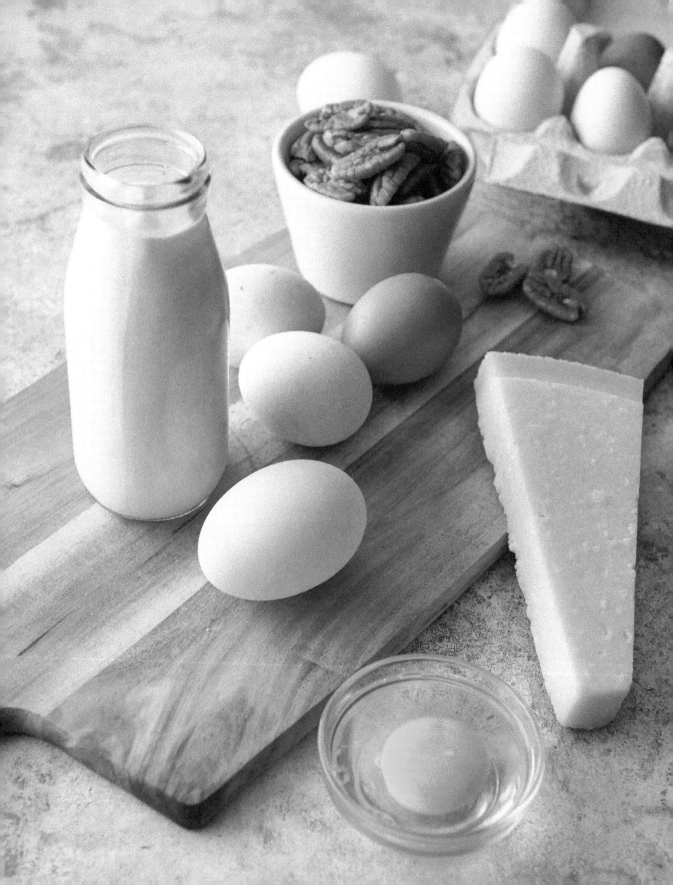

Measurement Conversions

	US STANDARD	US STANDARD (OUNCES)	METRIC (APPROXIMATE)	OVEN TEMPERATURES	
				F°	C°
VOLUME EQUIVALENTS (LIQUID)	2 tablespoons	1 fl. oz.	30 mL		
	¼ cup	2 fl. oz.	60 mL	250°F	120°F
	½ cup	4 fl. oz.	120 mL	300°F	150°C
	1 cup	8 fl. oz.	240 mL	325°F	180°C
	1½ cups	12 fl. oz.	355 mL	375°F	190°C
	2 cups or 1 pint	16 fl. oz.	475 mL	400°F	200°C
	4 cups or 1 quart	32 fl. oz.	1 L	425°F	220°C
	1 gallon	128 fl. oz.	4 L	450°F	230°C
VOLUME EQUIVALENTS (DRY)	⅛ teaspoon	—	0.5 mL		
	¼ teaspoon	—	1 mL		
	½ teaspoon	—	2 mL		
	¾ teaspoon	—	4 mL		
	1 teaspoon	—	5 mL		
	1 tablespoon	—	15 mL		
	¼ cup	—	59 mL		
	⅓ cup	—	79 mL		
	½ cup	—	118 mL		
	⅔ cup	—	156 mL		
	¾ cup	—	177 mL		
	1 cup	—	235 mL		
	2 cups or 1 pint	—	475 mL		
	3 cups	—	700 mL		
	4 cups or 1 quart	—	1 L		
	½ gallon	—	2 L		
	1 gallon	—	4 L		
WEIGHT EQUIVALENTS	½ ounce	—	15 g		
	1 ounce	—	30 g		
	2 ounces	—	60 g		
	4 ounces	—	115 g		
	8 ounces	—	225 g		
	12 ounces	—	340 g		
	16 ounces or 1 pound	—	455 g		

Keto Resources

Here are some keto resources that got me started on my journey. I'm including them here in case they're helpful for you, too.

Podcasts and Podcast Episodes

The Adam Corolla Show (There are several episodes with Vinnie Tortorich as a recurring guest.)

Fitness Confidential with Vinnie Tortorich

The Joe Rogan Experience (There have been many episodes that discuss keto.)

Keto for Normies

The Paleo Solution Podcast with Robb Wolf

STEM-Talk (Episode 87: Dom D'Agostino reflects on his 10 years of research into ketogenic nutrition.)

Websites and Youtube Channels

Jason Wittrock's YouTube channel

ketonutrition.org

marksdailyapple.com

paleochef.com

Books

The Big Fat Surprise: Why Butter, Meat and Cheese Belong in a Healthy Diet by Nina Teicholz

Eat Bacon Don't Jog by Grant Petersen

Eat Happy by Anna Vocino

Good Calories, Bad Calories: Fats, Carbs, and the Controversial Science of Diet and Health by Gary Taubes

The Ketogenic Cookbook by Jimmy Moore and Maria Emmerich

Why We Get Fat: And What to Do About It by Gary Taubes

Documentaries

Cereal Killers

FAT

Fed Up

The Magic Pill

Recipe Index

Index

Acknowledgments

Big shocker, but first I'd like to thank my mom. I know that is to be expected from one of the world's most famous mamma's boys, but for this book, my mom really is to thank. Obviously for being the best and most loving mom in the world, but more importantly, she's the greatest cook I've ever met. All of my mom's dishes are made from love, precision, and mad traditional Sicilian skill. I've been watching her cook amazing dishes my entire life. In the kitchen, she taught me that less is more. I've watched her make the most amazing dishes by always keeping it simple and adding in a few of her signature ingredients. I've applied all of her cooking principles to my keto dishes, and the results are the perfect blend of my low-carb cuisine mixed with mamma Paola's flare. To this day I still call my mom to ask her questions while I am cooking, like, "Ma, how do I heat the butter without melting it completely?" or "Ma, how do I broil my keto pizza dough so it cooks evenly?" She's always there for me, and now I'm here to share her skills with the rest of the world through my food.

Thank you to all the low-carb/high-fat influencers and resources who have inspired me along the way. Whether it was through podcasts, documentaries, books, or social media, I've learned so much from these amazing people who have been brave enough to go against the Standard American Diet and spread the unpopular truth about our heath and food system. I've always been worried that these scholars, doctors, nutritionists, and so on would not be receptive to a fist-pumping reality star being a keto influencer, but they have been nothing but kind, helpful, and grateful that I am spreading the word to the best of my abilities.

Thank you to all of my fans and followers on social media. I love all of you. I have to pinch myself every day from the disbelief that I actually have fans. But I'm especially grateful for those who have followed my @ketoguido Instagram page. I started that page as a side passion because I didn't want to annoy people on my @vinnyguadagnino page with photos of food, clips from documentaries and podcasts, or keto research articles. As of the printing of this book, that page now has around 800k followers (and by the time you're reading this, I hope even more) from people who are highly engaged, genuinely interested in my journey, and want to live a healthier life. I'm not an expert, but through @ketoguido I've been able to be a starting point for thousands of people who can then do more research on their own and learn from the real professionals. Every day I get thankful messages from followers, and I've even had some people lose hundreds of pounds just from becoming aware of this way of life. You give me meaning, and have made me realize that one of my life's purposes is to help people get healthier by using my spotlight. I will continue to help whoever I can, however I can, with this book and all of my platforms.

Thank you to all of my agents at ICM. I'd especially like to thank Matt Sorger, Heather Karpas, and Zoe Sandler. It's been a long road of trying to get this book written with multiple doors shut in our face. But with your help and belief in me, we found a way to make it happen and I am forever grateful.

Thank you to Pippa White and Callisto Media for publishing this book. You gave a silly reality star a chance at writing something that is fun but still spreads a serious message and shares this passion of mine. You've been a pleasure to work with.

Thank you also to Sam Greenspan, Michelle Anderson, Amy Treadwell, Elizabeth Castoria, Vanessa Putt, Jami Spittler, Kristine Brogno, Amy Burditt, Ashley Polikoff, Riley Hoffman, and Kim Ciabattari, who helped make this book a reality.

I'd like to thank the people who are responsible for keeping me in the spotlight and giving me this platform in the first place. The executive producers of *Jersey Shore*, SallyAnn Salsano and Jackie French, without you the world wouldn't have seen me drunkenly pull cheese and pepperoni off of my pizza, which introduced my keto ways to the world. You continue to let the Keto Guido shine through television. Everyone else at MTV and 495 productions that help and support me, I thank you as well.

Lastly, I'd like to thank my BFF, Pauly D, for yelling "Wake up, Keto Guido!" on season one of *Jersey Shore Family Vacation*. It is through your annoying screaming that the Keto Guido now has a catchphrase.

About the Author

Vinny Guadagnino rose to fame on MTV's *Jersey Shore*, which ran for six seasons and is the highest rated series in MTV's history. Vinny can now be seen in the reunion show, *Jersey Shore Family Vacation*. He is the bestselling author of *Control the Crazy: My Plan to Stop Stressing, Avoid Drama, and Maintain Inner Cool*, and is an advocate for mental health with teens and college students. An Honors graduate from CUNY College of Staten Island, Vinny lives in Staten Island, New York.